Wanted: The #1 Opioid Prescription Forger & Doctor Shopper

True Stories of Surviving 20 Years of Opioid Addiction

☞ **PART I – The Stories** ☜

Keith "Woody" LaPointe

Wanted: The #1 Opioid Prescription Forger & Doctor Shopper

True Stories of Surviving 20 Years of Opioid Addiction

☞ **PART I – The Stories** ☜

Copyright © 2020 by Keith LaPointe & R. L. Boyington

R. L. Boyington, Editor & Publisher

This is a work of non-fiction. Names and locations have been changed to protect the innocent, but characters and events are real.

Cover photograph—clockwise, from top left: generics for Norco, Vicodin, and Lortab, [Hydrocodone-Acetaminophen 10-325; Hydrocodone-Acetaminophen 5-325; and Hydrocodone-Acetaminophen 5-325].

—From a reader—

—about my experience with morphine. On the very first day in hospital, the doctors told me that due to my medication allergies, I would receive morphine. It was explained that I would be able to control my dose and that I would need to detox later.

I had strong reactions to the drug while hospitalized. I felt fine but was very short-fused (which I did not notice) and had trouble remembering and focusing. A friend visiting me told the nurses that my behavior was not normal and advised me to lower the dosage by trying to accept some discomfort, which I did.

Even with the lower dosage, the memory troubles meant I could follow a conversation, interact with someone, and forget five minutes later what we both said. I wrote notes to help—but later was not able to decipher them. LOL

When I returned home, I lowered the dosage again and developed bizarre reactions: hallucinations, day-dreaming, cold sweats, uncontrollable anger, panic attacks, insomnia. I spent nearly two weeks in this state, fighting to regain some control.

So, when my doctor told me it was time to end the morphine completely, we were both confident that in one week, I could do it painlessly. Ah! What a joke. I had the same strong reactions as earlier when I only lowered the dosage.

This experience gave me solid respect for drug addicts trying to fight drugs. I took them under medical control and for no more than four or five months. It was enough to get used to them and for my body to long for them. I gave all the remaining doses to my doctor, even when she told me I could keep some of them. I am not surprised that it can take months to have drugs entirely gone from your system!

—V. Barry

—Editor's Note—

Most of the stories recalled in this memoir were dictated into a smartphone while the author, Keith LaPointe, was driving a steel-laden big rig to and from New York City. From a faithful type-written transcription of those records, and from text messages exchanged between the author and the editor, comes this story of a life of addiction and recovery—and readdiction. The editor has tried to truthfully retain the voice of the author throughout, making only minor changes and adjustments in punctuation and grammar that would not be obvious in the spoken record. The editor has also tried to conceal, where appropriate, the identities of people involved and of particular locations.

—**Contents**—

5—Editor's Note

9—a long and needed rest

10—vitamins or something harmless

13—everybody knows everybody

15—everyone wants to be your friend

17—I'm out of here

18—end of the line

20—pane in your eye

23—what we did in 1973

27—forging a prescription

29—more of an asset than a liability

30—make up a social security number

32—me with all the garb on

34—the three stooges

36—the way it actually was

37—direct me to the ER

38—old and ready to retire

40—one of a kind

42—to be clean

43—my entire body was on fire

45—nothing but a blur

47—an intelligent addict

49—old enough for me

51—under surveillance

53—for the sake of my art

55—all of these favors

57—everyone did it

59—piss for probation

61—with these regrets

63—intervention

65—grateful

66—just to survive

67—being clean

69—another finely orchestrated and executed plan

70—her son was a junkie

75—getting my shit together

77—how beautiful life is

79—happily married

80—shadow on the wall

82—like a thief in the night

85—Dexedrine

88—the Narcan Challenge

90—About the Author

—"a long and needed rest"—

I forged prescriptions and doctor-shopped for 20 years—every single day. At work, at home, and yes, even on vacation. I had to. For both my wife and myself to not get sick. And to be able to pay our bills. It was a burden that broke me many, many times, causing depression and anxiety, fear of going to jail and not being able to provide for my family, and stress over my wife's addiction. I suffered this way all the time. It was too much weight to carry. Even to re-live the story is an unpleasant reminder. But I need to try to make it worth something to my family and to those who might otherwise end up living this kind of life of addiction.

I destroyed my reputation as a trusted person and friend. All thrown away while still trying to hold on to my pride and dignity. And my family. It was a 20-year war. I had to either help the police as an informant or go to prison and abandon my family. When I finally had had enough of being so mentally and physically exhausted and just couldn't fight any longer, I gave up and went to prison, sentenced to four years. I only did 30 months, but it became a long and needed rest.

Jail saved my life.

Sadly, I lost my dad while I was incarcerated, never being able to say goodbye or show him how I had finally straightened up at the age of 48. I also lost all of my material possessions—car, furniture, money. And friends. I had to start life all over again.

—"vitamins or something harmless"—

Everyone I knew, all my friends, were doing Speed and getting it from some Ivy League student. We would do this stuff called Bathtub Speed, or whatever the chemistry majors at college mixed up. We took anything that we got our hands on. Ate it. Snorted it.

When my wife got pregnant, we left my mom's, where we had been staying after a move from Florida, and moved in with my wife's mother. My wife breastfed our son, who miraculously was not born addicted. About this time, I had a job filling vending machines for UTech in East W. They soon transferred me to M., doing the same work. As a result of the transfer, we needed to move yet again—three times in a row.

Just before this last move, I hooked up with the person that became my pot dealer. He was also selling pills, and I was taking them. At first, I would only take some of them and sell just enough to pay for what I owed him for the bags of pills. He would bring over shopping bags(!) filled with an assortment of bottles of pills. This was when *drugs were drugs*. Quaalude, Percobarb, Seconal, Biphetamine or Black Beauties (Adderall), Demerol, Tuinal, Nembutal, Dilaudid, Percodan, Percocet, and on and on and on.

This guy, the pot dealer, called me one night and told me of people he knew who would break into pharmacies—by entering through the roof! This was before good alarm systems and safes had come into everyday use. And this I would remember.

I would sell only to the people I got high with and a few other people I knew from around town. At that time, I would sell the pills cheap: $2 to $2.59 a pill. This went on for roughly six months. Then I met this girl who worked at a local pharmacy, and she happened to like pot. I would trade her a $10 bag of weed, a quarter ounce at the time, for a bottle of Percodan. She would stuff a 100-count bottle with as many pills as she could. She continued to be my source of Percodan for a few months—until she lost her job.

My connections, my sources, had now dried up. That's when I, and the friends that I sold to, took matters into our own hands.

We began by calling in prescriptions. We would call in an emergency order for pills. One person who knew all the pharmaceutical lingo would call the pharmacy from a nearby phone booth. Meanwhile, another person would go into the pharmacy, listen to the pharmacist on the phone talking with our friend outside, while pretending to look for vitamins or something harmless. The pharmacist would always repeat, out loud, what the phone booth "doctor" was calling in, 30 tablets of Percocet, or whatever. If the pharmacist didn't immediately pick up the phone and call back the actual patient, or the police, we knew it was alright to approach and pick up the prescription. The laws were much laxer in those days. So, we'd wait for about half an hour and send in a third person to pick up the prescription.

My wife and I were now cleaning homes for a living. One day, while we were cleaning a doctor's house, we found a few loose, blank prescription sheets from Hospice. I took them. I called the kid who used to run a phone-in scam with us because he knew the pharmaceutical lingo. I asked him if he could use the prescriptions I had found. He said, "Absolutely!" That's when I learned how to "write scripts"—that is, how to forge prescriptions. We began with a few pharmacies, and none of them would fill the order. So, we called it quits for the day. The next day I tried again, this time at a local pharmacy. The prescription I forged was for 50 pills of Percocet. The pharmacist filled it. Eureka, I was in!

My wife and I became pretty well addicted to opioids. We just used the pills we got, never sold them. But feeding our addiction was becoming a fulltime job in itself. So, I did less work and more prescription fraud, and doctor shopping. And, I needed to start selling pills if I wanted to supplement our income.

The buddy who ran the phone-in scam with us taught me about doctor shopping. You go to the doctor and tell them, "My testicles hurt," he suggested. Because if you tell them your back or legs hurt, they end up giving you muscle relaxers. We were only after the opioids. So, I would go to urologists and tell them, "I was riding a bike with my son," you know, the family man angle, "when suddenly the chain snapped, and I landed on the crossbar." The doctor would squirm and write a script for

Percodan or Percocet. And an antibiotic. And maybe a scrotal support. Yeah sure, as if I'd buy the scrotal support. I needed all the money for the scripts.

After I saw how easy it was, I increased my doctor shopping. So much so that I ended up running out of local doctors to see. That's when I decided to switch up the *ailment*. Another buddy of mine suggested a doctor in New H. he knew that gave out pills. Only one problem. He was a proctologist. Before long, here I was bent over his table, looking around, trying to take my mind off the fact that I was about to have a finger shoved up my asshole. All I could see were hoses and all kinds of instruments lying around the room, and I'm thinking to myself, "Jesus Christ, what have I gotten into?" Soon the doc started running hoses from the sink, setting up instruments, and I was getting pretty embarrassed. There was nothing wrong with me, but I had to play the part of the sick patient. The worst part was that the nurse was a young and pretty girl. I walked out with a sore ass and only 10 Percocet!

—"everybody knows everybody"—

There were good times, you know, with some of the users I went around with. We would stop at a strip joint after we finished getting our scripts or after the pharmacies had closed, and if we had done well, life was good. At the strip club, we would give the girls pills instead of money.

I remember one time in the town of W., we'd just got all these pills, and I was counting them to divide them up. There were three of us, me and two other guys in the car. I was in the passenger side front seat, and there was this chick walking down the sidewalk, so we whistled. There was a detective car behind us which we hadn't noticed, and all of a sudden, they put on their lights and pulled us over. Two cops came up, one on the driver's side, and one went to my side. Now, the pills were in my lap, and I hadn't had time to put them away. The cop goes, "Get out of the car." I said, "What for?" He said, "Just get out of the car," and I said, "Why do you want us out of the car?" He said we fit the description of some robbers that had just robbed a store. I think they were just busting our balls because as it ended up, I refused to get out of the car, nobody got out of the car, and the cops just left. It was one of the many weird things that happened out on the road doing scripts.

There was another time with those same two guys when we tried to rob a pharmacy by getting in through the roof. Thanks for the idea, pot dealer! The two guys climbed up. But not me. It was pretty high up, *and* I was too heavy. They were going to get through the roof with hatchets and pry bars. I was watching out when I saw a cop coming down the street, and I yelled, "Cop!" And one of the kids said to the other, "Jump!" But he wouldn't. So, the first one pushed him, and the kid turned completely over in the air and grabbed the gutter. He was like a cat. They ended up running off into the woods. I tried to follow but didn't make it. I hit a tree. So, there I was, laying there like a slug on the side of the parking lot near the woods. If the cop had pulled back there, he would have seen me. The other two were well into the woods when suddenly I hear this splash. They had fallen into a river!

Lucky for us, the cop left, and the guys came out of the woods soaked. That was the end of that. All our break-in tools were left behind on the roof of the pharmacy.

One of the things that I used to do in the town where we were doing scripts was to make use of phone booths (when they had phone booths). This was in the early '80s. Some of the booths would have the white customer pages. We would rip out these pages and use these names and addresses as patients in our scripts. This was before computers, so the pharmacists would look up the names and addresses in the phone book to see if they matched. Sometimes you would have to write the patient information on your wrists so you could remember the name you were using and just hope that the pharmacist didn't personally know the patient you were using. With larger cities, you could just pick a patient's name and address and be pretty sure you wouldn't get caught. But with a smaller town, everybody knows everybody.

—"everyone wants to be your friend"—

When I was on the Methadone program, I was standing in line one day and talking to this dude. Behind us in line was this guy with makeup on. He was a real freak, a good kid though. The guy I was talking with said, "Look at that fag," and I said, "You know what, I bet he gets more pussy than both of us. Don't make fun of the kid because he dresses like that." As it turns out, me and the kid that dressed up all girly became friends. He was a musician, a lead singer in a band and his name was Johnny. He wore fishnet stockings. This kid was nuts.

One time, Johnny had to go to this gig, and he was at my home, dyeing his hair pink. I said I was going to nod off for a while. He also napped on my couch. Later, I found his fucking hair dye all over the white pillow on my couch. It was ruined, and my towels too. Well, we went on to this gig in W., and he said he wanted me to be the band's manager, but all I wanted to do was sell drugs to the band. Johnny had business cards made up and everything. His band had a contract with RCA at one time. They were pretty big for a local band. Vanilla Ice was at that gig I mentioned, so we all got pictures with him. He was nothing at the time. The thing is, the kid in the band was real punk crazy shit. He had a massive scar across his chest where, during one gig, someone had thrown a broken bottle at him because he always tried to one-up his audience. He spat on the crowd, and they spat on him. It was fucking nuts man. The bottle left this huge scar. He was just one of the characters that I met during all this crazy drug shit. I sent him into a few pharmacies. He liked Xanax; that's what he was into. Some of the girls that he would date were just beautiful, man. It was fucking nuts.

I brought Johnny out to the strip joints once in West H., it was after the gig in W., and all the chicks were looking at him wearing fishnet stockings and short shorts. It was just another crazy night on drugs.

This kid had balls. That is why I had respect for him. He didn't care the fuck about nothing. You have to have a lot of guts to walk around like that, man, high heels, fishnets, pink hair. Jesus Christ. All the strippers liked him. I got posters of him at my house. This kid backed up a lot of bands in the '80s, like Quiet Riot, groups like that. I wasn't into those bands, and he was younger than me and into head-banging stuff, punk, the new rock during the '80s. Johnny had a drug problem and never made it real big.

    The one thing about being involved with drugs, about having pills, is that everyone wants to be your friend. But I'll tell you something. You won't be meeting any fucking scholars or very nice people. Most of them are low-lifes, degenerates, thieves, scoundrels. They would come to my house, and I would catch them trying to steal something. I would have to put a knife to their throat and say, "If you do it again, I will fucking kill you," and I'd never let them back in the house again.

—"I'm out of here"—

Besides all the drug stuff going on in my life back in the '70s, there was a lot of family shit, too. Not all of it drug and alcohol-related. For example, a few days after my brother shot his wife and then himself (unsuccessfully) with a 12-gauge shotgun, me, my mom and dad had to go clean out my brother's house. My brother's wife's parents came over and took her things out. But we had to do the rest of the cleaning. My mom rolled up the carpet where my sister-in-law had died. I don't think they allow families to do that nowadays. By rights, we should have just left it, but things were different back in 1976. I was helping my parents pack things up when I removed a picture hanging on the wall. But when I lifted it up, I heard this dink, dink, dink of something hitting the floor. I bent down and picked up what turned out to be two of my brother's teeth and part of his jawbone, blown away in his suicide attempt. I turned to my mother and said, "I'm out of here." And I left. I must have been in shock.

Later, I went up to the state mental hospital almost every week to visit my brother. One of my first friends with whom I started getting high, Louie, was also there. He said that all of my problems started with my father. Louie wore these glasses that looked like coke bottles. He said all *his* problems were his eyes. He was flipping out, so I had to stop hanging around him because he was fucking with my head. I always saw people up at the hospital that I used to get high with. When I was going up there, I was smoking Angel Dust, and I told my brother I had to get out of there—it seemed like a freak show, people with scars on their heads from lobotomies, people falling on the floor, having seizures. It wasn't very nice.

—"end of the line"—

To begin at the beginning. I first started getting high at the age of 15, when my older brother came home from the Vietnam War. He passed me a joint while we were riding in his car. It shocked and scared me.

Before that, I had played sports—basketball, baseball, and football. That all ended when I started getting high. While getting high with my brother, I also began to hang around other kids who got high. During the '70s, all kinds of drugs were available. I did them all.

Except for heroin. Heroin was taboo. Heroin meant the end of the line.

So, I started with pot in 1971, then hashish, hash oil, and of course, alcohol. Then an assortment of pills: Valium, "THC" tablets (but who knows what it really was; some people said horse tranquilizer). Then White Crosses, LSD, Mescaline, Cocaine, Quaaludes, and even Nitrous Oxide once from a tank. In 1975 I took my first Percodan. Then Cocaine came around, and so did different types of Speed, then Angel Dust in 1977, along with another dust that we snorted. Real potent stuff. Put you right into the ozone. I wouldn't let my wife (girlfriend at the time) touch either it or Angel Dust. Much too powerful. And Speed, which was coming out of the nearby college, I was told, where my buddy was getting it.

Angel Dust [Phencyclidine, or PCP] was introduced to me by two deaf kids I worked with while building pallets. They had just moved back to N. B. from California, where they had gotten it. It was sprayed on mint leaves, and they had about an ounce of it. It was so strong that when you rolled a joint, you only needed to roll enough to be the size of a nail used to join a 2 x 4 piece of wood. Very little, but that would be enough to get four people really high.

About that time, my cousin DJ came back into my life, now that he had started to get high, but only on weed, no Cocaine yet. It was March 1978, and I was at the point where I knew that I was going to be dead very soon if I didn't get out of the whole drug scene. I called my uncle RJ in Florida and asked him if I could come down and get clean and work with him for a while. He said no problem, Keith. While I was in Florida, I told my fiancée that I needed to get right in my head, and I would send for her once I found a place for us to live. She was just getting ready to graduate from a school of business, and I asked my cousin to watch out for her.

I spent a month working with my uncle. He made me save all the money I made, only letting me buy cigarettes. Everything else he took care of. Food, a place to live, pot to smoke. He had a shrub of pot plants the length of his house. They looked like hedges. LOL. But by 3 weeks into being away from my fiancée, I missed her terribly, and so asked her to marry me when I came back home. Between my mother, my fiancée and her mother, and my sister—they had everything ready for me to step into a tuxedo and say I DO.

That first time I got high wasn't because I wanted to. In 1971 more than half of my friends were smoking pot, sniffing glue, and stealing pills from their parents' medicine cabinets. I was asked to join in but never pressured to do so. It took someone very close to me that I had looked up to my whole life. My older brother. He had just come home a Marine. We were close, and he would take me with him riding around even though he was 7 years older than me. One day we went to Dunkin Donuts and had coffee. He had a crush on the girl that worked there and eventually married. While we were driving back home to our parents' house, he took a joint out of his top shirt pocket and lit it up. It made me feel nervous and uncomfortable, then he passed it to me. I did smoke cigarettes but never pot or any other drugs. Because I looked up to and respected my brother, I took a hit. He dropped me off at the house, and I walked straight to the bathroom and puked, then into the bedroom, and fell face down on the bed. We told our parents that I had too much coffee and got sick.

I was finally able to relate to the stoners and heads who did drugs. And, to have my older brother think that I was cool, and ready to hang out with him. I continued getting high.

—"pane in your eye"—

I was hanging around with Jim, the kid who first turned me on to LSD, in the center of the town where we both lived. We had a mutual friend who had moved out to New Mexico. This friend of ours came back to visit his family and also brought back some LSD. The name of the Acid was Window Pane. I had never done this kind of Acid before. I tripped only 10 times in my entire life; this was probably the 3rd time. This particular LSD looked like a piece of scotch tape. It was approximately 1/8-inch square and see-through clear. We only had one hit, one dose of it, so we cut it in half with a razor blade. Now before we took the LSD, or "dropped Acid" as it is called, my buddy said that you're supposed to do Window Pane in your eye. Yeah, that's right, *in your eye*, so that's what we did. Jim is the same friend who had turned all the stooges on to Acid the first time I had ever tried it (at age 17), which was also the first time I got arrested.

Jim had done a lot of LSD already by his 22nd year of life. He really enjoyed it. Anyway, we put the Window Pane in the corner of our eyes, and within a half-hour, we were tripping. But the shit was really irritating my eye, and if you're tripping, it seems like the irritation is ten times worse than it should be.

So there we were, me and Jim doing Acid at a house that belonged to another friend who had gotten into a horrible car accident a year earlier. This friend had been in a coma for a couple of months. He was so fucked up from the accident that his face had to have extensive reconstructive surgery, and one of his legs ended up being 4 inches shorter than the other. By rights, he shouldn't have been alive; but he was, barely. So, there we were, tripping on Acid and also getting high on some pot. The kid whose house it was had a 4-foot hookah pipe that we were smoking out of. The bowl was so big that he had to put a record album over the top of the bowl so it would stay lit. It had maybe 6 hoses for people to smoke from, but it was just the three of us, and two of us were now tripping like crazy.

The sister of the kid who was in the accident was an artist and had covered the walls in fluorescent colored paint with zigzag patterns and a lot of hippie flowers and crazy designs. When you're tripping, it's all a bit too much at times, but the craziest part for me was when I would look at the kid who was in the car accident, he started to look like a fucking spider. I swear to God, a fucking long-legged spider. I'd look at Jim, who was also tripping, and we would just start laughing as if we knew what the other was thinking. That's how LSD works. And with the kid all fucked up from the 4-inch heel on his boot and all the reconstruction surgery done on his face with one glass eye and just being a real mess, God forgive me for this, but between dragging his gimp leg around and the rest of his deformities, he was a spider to me, so I said to Jim, I got to get the fuck outta here, man.

Jim and I left on foot, neither of us had a car at the time, and we walked about 3 miles back to the center of our home town. While we were sitting on a bench, a cop walked up the street from the police department only 100 yards away and stood across the street, just standing there watching us. We were laughing at him, and we left and began to walk to my buddy's home, his parents' house. I remember walking up a hill in the middle of the street, when I just collapsed and told Jim that I couldn't go on, that I couldn't breathe. He was laughing at me, said get up we're almost there. We eventually made it.

Jim was a hippie guitar-playing dude, my buddy who did the LSD with me, and he was playing his folk guitar in the kitchen while I was in the bathroom looking in the mirror at my swollen uvula. I felt like I was suffocating from it being so swollen. Meanwhile, my buddy was playing Cat Stevens in the kitchen, and I was dying in the bathroom, looking at my swollen uvula in the mirror. What a trip that was.

The kid with the gimp died a couple of years later. The gimp was with a girl in a small MG sports car. The girl was giving him oral sex when he hit a tree. She was all gimped out, too, but sued him for a lot of money.

My buddy Jim, with the Acid, ended up in a wheelchair from a dirty needle or an infection from a dirty syringe. He died in the late '90s.

One of the kids that did Acid with me the first time has had AIDS for about 20 years but is at least still alive. He was a junkie, did needles.

The other kid that had done Acid for the first time with me lives in Florida and has problems with Crack.

Most of the people who I grew up getting high with are all dead. That's the usual ending with drugs, an early death. It's a sad scourge of today's lifestyle, and now it's getting even worse with the Oxycodone type drugs.

I consider myself a conservative drug abuser, just enough to not be sick and not enough to be shit faced. Or dead.

I'm lucky to be alive.

—"what we did in 1973"—

Not one thing in my life came easy from the time I started doing drugs, from the first joint to the last pill.

When I was 17, I tried LSD for the first time. It was also the first time I was arrested. Me and four buddies were hanging out at the local beach, and one of my friends said, hey let's get high. We all said, yeah let's get high. So he reached into his pocket and took out a pack of cigarettes, and in the cellophane, he clawed out 4 tiny squares of white paper each a little over an eighth of an inch square. I had never even seen Acid before. He handed each of us a hit. Except for me and one of my friends who had also never done LSD. We split one hit. We cut it right through the center of the off-colored dot on the paper. We all dropped it on our tongues, and went for a ride.

Just drove around, that's what we did in 1973, popped in a Zeppelin 8-track tape and smoked some pot, and drank some beer. Since I was driving, I asked where does everyone want to go? Me and the friend that only did half a hit wanted to find some chicks, but the buddy that had the Acid suggested that we go down to the quarry. The quarry is famous for its pink granite, one of only a couple of sources of pink granite in the world. The base of the Statue of Liberty has pink granite from there, as well as the base of the Brooklyn Bridge and some other famous structures in New York City. So, we headed to the quarry. But around the back, there was an unused entrance that my buddy knew about.

There was a cable blocking the grass-covered road, but it was laying on the ground, so I drove over it. A half-mile into the woods, we came upon a massive hole in the ground. And the end of the road. I turned the car around and turned off the engine. There was a huge building with a glass front for observation of the quarry. The kid with the Acid started to throw rocks at the glass, and not long after, we all joined in throwing rocks. About this time, it began to get dark. There we were, laughing and drinking and smoking pot when, all of a sudden, a pickup truck came barreling up the grass road, and we all turned and ran into the woods.

But there was a hill about 6 feet high, and me and another kid couldn't climb it, so we stood motionless. Now I drove a 1962 Nova 2-door, and the passenger side door wouldn't open until Bubba, one of the quarry workers, ripped it open. The workers looked around and got back into the pickup truck and drove back down the road that we all came in on. I could have sworn that they heard my heart pounding out of my chest, and being that we were all tripping on Acid, everything was very surreal. We jumped into the car to get the fuck outta there. That was the plan anyway. As we approached the two poles where the cable had been on the ground, it was now hooked up. I started to drive under it when, without warning, patrol car lights went on. My friend in the back seat said everyone give me your pot and pipes, I'm going to run. We all handed our paraphernalia to him, but the two huge Bubbas were walking up to the car. I told my friend not to run. We ended up stashing the pot and pipes under the front seat.

Now the cops and the two big guys were walking to the car, and the big Bubba type dude pulled open the broken passenger door again, and we all got out of the car. We were arrested and my vehicle was towed. We were really tripping off the Acid. We were fingerprinted and booked.

This was a brand-new police station, and as I was being led to the cell, I heard Keeiitthh in a high-pitched weaselly voice. A friend of ours, he was the first person to be locked up in the new jail. For me, it was the first time on LSD, the first time being arrested and the second person in the new jail cell. Not a good night.

The cop at the desk was a friend of my family, my dad played poker with occasionally. Now my friend that had the Acid was a real nut and fun to get high with. He had tripped well over 500 times but bragged of it being 1000 times. They used to call him FLY because he was always buzzed, like in the song by the group AMERICA, a fly with a buzz. Now I could see him a few cells down and he was a real skinny dude about 6' 2" tall. He was lying across the cell bars with his feet sticking out of the bars. His elbow was sticking out of the other bars as if he was reclining like you'd lie on your side with your head resting on your hand propped up by your elbow. Nothing ever bothered this kid. Nothing, a real free spirit, a true hippie.

The cops searched us and took our shoelaces when we got put into the jail cell, but they didn't get my friend's penknife that was on his belt loop. We passed it on, and we carved our names on those new cell walls. They kept us there for about 8 to 10 hours, I really don't know how long, until we stopped tripping. The whole trip was spent in jail.

The cop asked us who to call. My mom came down to bond me out. She ended up bonding three of us out. One kid got out early because his father had connections. Two of my buddies' parents would have just left them in there. My mom didn't realize that if even one of them didn't show up at court, she could have lost her home because that is what she had for collateral. She was real pissed off because the so-called friend of her and my father didn't make her aware of that part.

We all got charged with criminal mischief and trespassing. I also got charged for possession of pot. The police found a bag of pot seeds in my glove compartment. But they never found the weed or pipes that we had stashed under the front seat. We all had to pay $21 for the broken windows and got 1-year probation.

Exactly 1 month later, I was arrested for possession of marijuana and fireworks. I went back to the same judge who had just recently sentenced us, and of course, me being a juvenile, my parents had to be present at both court cases. After the first bust, my father said that if I ever got arrested again, don't call him or my mom to bond me out. So, this second time I called my older brother, and he came down to the same police department to get me out.

I didn't tell my parents that I had been arrested a second time until we had a family get-together. The whole family was there, so I thought that would be a good time to tell my dad. He exploded, oh man, he also had to go back to court with me. My mother always came even though I was embarrassed to go with my mommy, LOL, but she insisted. Anyway, the judge said talk to your probation officer, and I'll go by his recommendation. My probation officer said that if I can beat the charge, okay, so the next court date, I told the judge what he said, and I received a $50 fine for the bag of pot and $10 for the fireworks, and that was it.

I didn't get arrested again until it was for obtaining drugs with a forged prescription … in 1983. That was 9 years with no probation.

Following that, I was on probation or parole until 2007. That's what drugs got me—never ever free from drugs and the state. I've been owned by both for my entire adult life. Sad what drugs have done to me and millions of other people who wished to have been free of addiction. We didn't start out to be slaves to drugs, but the drugs have a different idea of what is going to happen with your life.

—"forging a prescription"—

The very first prescription paper I ever forged and used was Hospice care paper. The hospital was only ½ mile away from my house. But Hospice was like the VA hospitals, where the majority of the doctors were *floaters*, doctors who worked in multiple hospitals or had privileges in different hospitals. At the time, my wife and I cleaned houses for a living. We had a few doctors as clients, and some of them would bring the prescription pads home, probably being just too tired to remember to leave them at the hospital at the end of their shifts. I found a few loose prescription papers on a counter in one of the houses, so I took a couple. I showed my buddy who would play the doctor when we called into the pharmacies to get the drugs. He said, yeah, we can try them. That night we did, but no pharmacy would fill it for us, so I took it back home to use as a template for writing more scripts.

That was one of the ways of forging a prescription. There are many variations, and rules for each drug. Prescriptions are all written in Latin from the beginning of time as being part of the doctor's mystique. Or so that we common folk don't know what's going on. Once you write a script and date it, it needs to be filled that day, especially if it's a Schedule II narcotic because of the tight control over those drugs. If you bring it to a pharmacy and they write on it, for example, your birthday, address, telephone number, and especially if they stamp it with the store's own stamp, it's ruined for other pharmacies. It puts up a red flag as to why it wasn't filled at that first pharmacy. It is frowned upon by other pharmacies as not being a legitimate prescription, or it would have been filled.

So now I had a couple of the Hospice papers when I, my wife, and son were at her family's house for dinner. My wife and I were sick from not having recently taken Percocet. I had brought one of the prescription papers with me in case I found the nerve to go by myself and try to have it filled. I had never done a forged prescription before. We, the group of buddies, had called drugs in but never used a prescription paper. So, I took a ride out to one town away, and sat in front of the CVS pharmacy and was very nervous and wanted to just leave. I was scared shitless. I didn't want to do it, but being sick from withdrawals, it was either take a chance or go back to the in-laws and be even sicker. I went into the pharmacy and walked around until I finally got up the nerve to approach the pharmacy counter, and laid down the prescription. I am nervous just writing this now!

    The pharmacist asked me all the info, and don't forget it was written by me on a Hospice prescription blank. I had written it for 50 Percocet. I sat down and waited. Then the fake name I had written on the script was called. I went up, and the pharmacist told me how much I owed for the pills. I paid for it and was handed the bag. I felt like kissing the pharmacist. But didn't. I walked out with such relief and joy, surprised I wasn't floating. I got to the car that I had parked around the corner and drove to my in-law's house. My wife asked if it went down ok. I probably said no and told her that the cops were chasing me, knowing how I am and love the scared to elated look and mood change from her. I'm sure we had sex that night. That was my first store, the first prescription that I wrote and did on my own.

One year later, because that same pharmacy was my first and automatic favorite, it became the first pharmacy that I was arrested at. For obtaining drugs with a forged prescription and for attempting to obtain drugs with a forged prescription. First for both.

—"more of an asset than a liability"—

But of course, nothing comes free or cheap. I had to go to court a few times for each charge. I would have to give up or rat out someone for my statewide narcotics task force buddy. So that he could tell the prosecutor in whichever court I was going to, that I was more of an asset than a liability.

I swear to you the reader, I am being honest and straightforward here. Yeah, I know it sounds funny. This is the part of my story that brings me the greatest shame. Because I was respected by most of the people who knew me, and because being a rat meant that I lost a lot of respect for myself. Even though most of the people that knew me didn't hold it against me. I was and am a man of my word. I didn't do it just for me, but also for my wife and son. I couldn't leave them alone to fend for themselves. And with my wife being even more addicted than I was, she wasn't able to handle it when I tried to get clean by going into a program. She freaked out, cried out of fear of getting dope sick. Who would have taken care of our son? My parents offered to take care of him so that me and her could get clean, but she wasn't having any of that. I did what I had to do.

Like I said, I was going to multiple courts at the same time all year every year for the entire time I was forging prescriptions. I was doing so many scripts it was inevitable that I would get busted. For 1 out of 200-300 scripts, I was arrested either by being caught red-handed in the pharmacy or by a warrant based on photos being sent from one store to the next. If I was arrested in one town and used the same MO in the next, it only took a photo being sent between stores. Back when I started to forge prescriptions, there weren't any computers. Everything was done with typewriters, even police work. Computer networks put a dent in the prescription forgery business for sure.

—"make up a social security number"—

For the first couple of years that I was getting arrested for prescription fraud, the police didn't know how to charge me, whether it was a felony or a class B or A misdemeanor. They would just charge me for forgery, and for stealing the prescription paper. But in fact I would be photocopying some of them, so other times I would be charged with obtaining controlled drugs with a forged prescription. One time they even tried to get me for impersonating a doctor! It was quite the dilemma for them, LOL.

One police department, I think it was in W., counted all of the forged prescriptions the pharmacy had waiting for me on the counter when I went in one night. When the cops walked in and busted me, the pharmacist handed over a stack of scripts I had forged even though I had other people doing them right there with me. They charged me with multiple counts of obtaining, plus the one that I was going to do but was busted with. I was officially charged with attempting to obtain a controlled substance with a forged prescription. Anyway, they got me. Most of the charges carried the same penalties.

Days of prescription fraud and doctor shopping are over, what with computerized prescriptions, and the fact that all pharmacies are now interconnected. You can no longer go from doctor to doctor, at least with your own name. The doctors and pharmacies are also now asking for a driver's license or a picture ID. It makes it almost impossible now to get away with it. Even if you were able to get multiple doctors to write you scripts, you still have to get through the pharmacy's safety systems. Even if you pay cash and avoid an insurance company or state insurance, you still need the ID. Years ago, each independent pharmacy chain, for instance CVS, would only be connected to other CVS stores and not a different chain's store. But now all pharmacies have the technology to be connected to each other. I don't know if it's just for controlled substances or for all medications.

Not so long ago, my home state tried to pass a law that all Schedule II narcotics have to be sent via electronic prescription to the pharmacy and not written on paper. It failed to pass. It would have allowed the state to keep better track of which doctors are prescribing narcotics or over-prescribing them. And keep track of which patients are receiving Schedule II narcotics and have a good reason for taking them. One electronic ℞ copy would go to the pharmacy, another to the state DCP, and one stay in the doctor's office for their records. Doctors wanted instead to have the same system as New York and Rhode Island had back when I was forging prescriptions, as far back as the 1970s. Those states had the handwritten triplicate prescription pads, one copy to the state, one to the pharmacy, and the third stayed in the office or hospital. My state's doctors' association fought against the automated update because of the resulting watchful eye of the government.

In the early days of prescription fraud, you were very rarely asked for any form of identification either at the doctor's office or the pharmacy. Even hospitals didn't ask for an ID. So, I would just make up a social security number, address, and phone number. I didn't have to worry about cameras or closed-circuit TV. There weren't any. Otherwise, I would never have gotten away with it for so long. But like I said, you just can't get away with it anymore. The only thing that I had to worry about back then was the pharmacist picking up the phone or hitting a panic button under the counter. Even then, you could watch the faces of the people behind the counter for a nervous tic or a change of mood or reaction.

Another trick of the trade. I usually wrote the prescription in a woman's name. I conveniently wouldn't have her ID, and the person whose name it was written for would be in too much pain to walk in and get the prescription for herself. If I was sending a girl into the store, I would write it in a man's name so that it seemed like she was getting it for a father, brother, or husband. It was much more convenient that way.

—"me with all the garb on"—

Just when I feel I've said it all, something else comes up. I've got years and more years of drug-related memories.

One day I went out doing scripts by myself. I was driving around and ended up in the town of B. I had just banged out a script for 75 Percocet and was going to a Brooks chain pharmacy in this same town. This day I wore a getup I had used many times before. I had on a nice suit, with unassuming, gentle colors. A light pink shirt and a very nice Oscar de la Renta tie. And a cervical collar, plus a bandage on the bridge of my nose. There was red food coloring dripped onto the shirt and tie with a little under the dressing. I walked into the pharmacy and handed them the prescription and told them I needed some bandages and some Betadine solution. I was waiting for the script when I heard the rattle of keys, the kind of keys a cop wears on his belt. I carefully got up, peeked over the aisles, and started to walk out of the store.

The cops, three of them, were playing which aisle to go down. One of the cops stopped me and asked me to walk back to the pharmacist with him. There were two male cops and one female. The pharmacist identified me, and they walked me out to my car. They had already surrounded my vehicle with their squad cars. I don't know how they knew that it was mine, but they did. A detective came over to me with a piece of paper that he wanted me to sign, a consent to search my car. I signed it. Now the female cop was the one that searched my car. I had the pharmacy bag with 75 pills in it from the pharmacy I had just left and some other prescription paper. So, we got to the police department, and, before going into the cell, the detective asked me if the neck brace was necessary. I told him no, so I took it off. He came back to let me make my phone call. I called my wife, asked her to bring a friend of ours, and to stop at the pharmacy and get the car before they towed it. Next, the cop asked me if he could photograph me with all the garb on, cervical collar, the bandage on my nose, and so on. I humored him and agreed.

Now I was on probation at the time. I asked the cop if I could call a friend of mine. He asked who. That was my chance to mention my buddy, who was with the statewide narcotics task force, and I said his name. He told me, "I AM the narcotics task force." OK, I'm thinking, so no call. A couple of hours went by before my wife showed up. While the lady cop was tending to me—she was a really sweet girl—I mouthed to my wife, put a pill in your mouth, and kiss me. I asked the lady cop if I could get a kiss from my wife, and she said OK. I got the pill.

I was very depressed that night and was probably crying a bit. She, the cop, felt sorry for me. They never charged me for the pills or for doing the pharmacy before I was arrested. She had to have taken the whole bag with the pills in it, thank God. The male detective said that he should take my car because it's now contraband, and by law, they could have. It wasn't even a year old, a brand-new car, but my wife had possession of it, and he would have had to find it.

I didn't have bond money and didn't get to call my buddy with the pull. They put me back in handcuffs and brought me to the D. police department because the local jail wasn't equipped to hold prisoners overnight. We got there, and I had to wait there all night until the bail commissioner came in the morning to set everyone's bond price or let them out on a PTA (promise to appear) or bring us straight to court.

I got a PTA, my wife was waiting for me, and we went back home. I remember it was pouring rain that day, and the river was way up over the banks. I remember crying most of the way home from pure stress and being tired of everything. We finally got home, and now that I hadn't gotten any pills the night before, except for the ones that the lady cop took from me, I had to go into the house and grab more prescription paper and go right back out. So there I was just out of jail and within 2 hours back at it again. Never ending, never. I had to refocus and think of where to go and ended up going out to S., next to NYC, by myself again. I always went alone unless I had a person who I had trained.

—"the three stooges"—

There was this one time with the three stooges (the original gang who would call the drugs into the pharmacies instead of using prescription paper). How we would do it was the kid with all the knowledge of how it was done correctly over the telephone, he would play the part of the doctor. Another one of us would be the patient. There were no such things as cell phones or pagers, so either we would use a house phone or, more often, we used a phone booth. There was one in front of every strip mall or group of stores. So here's how we did it. One of us would be in the pharmacy near the counter where we could hear the phone ring and listen to the conversation between the so-called doctor and the pharmacist. If it was a pharmacy technician, they would put the "doctor" on hold and tell the pharmacist who it was that was calling.

We would know the name because it was our buddy calling. So, we would have our phony doctor making the call. The guy who listened in on the conversation, hung around long enough to make sure that the pharmacist didn't either call the police or try to call the doctor back. The lookout would hang out just a little while longer to make sure and listen to hear the safe being opened. Percocet or Percodan pills being counted. The tablets have a distinctive sound when being put into the bottle. Once we knew that it was ready for pick-up, we would send a different face in, one of us that the pharmacist hadn't seen yet. So, we would wait for a few minutes and then go in to pick up the drugs.

The one who played the doctor knew all of the jargon, in which order to prescribe the drugs, and to then give them the BNDD# (the narcotic dispensing number). At that time, in the late '70s and early '80s, you could only call in an emergency script of no more than twelve pills of Schedule II drugs. The doctor must send a paper prescription to the pharmacy as soon as possible for the records. The pharmacist needed to have the paper script for proof of dispensing, in case the DCP agents came in for an audit.

If you called in a cough syrup that contained a Schedule III drug, you didn't have to send a script in to cover the prescription. There was a pharmacy in E. H. that never had a safe but kept these drugs on a wooden shelf with a door and flimsy lock. I was curious about why most pharmacies used a safe while others didn't, so when I was summoned up to the state capital to talk to the DCP agents, I asked why. They told me that if a pharmacy is robbed, they are ordered by the DCP to get and use a safe.

Another time we stooges were calling in a prescription for Percodan, and one of us was in the store, and our fake doctor was right outside the store making the call. The store was right next to the DMV, so there was a lot of traffic. While the "doctor" was on the phone with the pharmacist, a few trucks were going by, and one blew his air horn. Well, the pharmacist could hear it, and he also heard the same truck horn on the "doctor's" phone. LOL. The pharmacist asked the doctor (our buddy) where he was making this call from! The pharmacist began to walk outside to look for the doctor. And there was our buddy, still on the phone. When the pharmacist yelled at him, he took off down the street. Needless to say, we didn't get any pills from that store.

—"the way it actually was"—

I am telling you everything the way it actually was. I'm 63 years old and really don't care about what people think of me as long as they know that I'm an honest asshole. LOL

—"direct me to the ER"—

In the town of M., about a half-hour's drive from home, I was once walking through the hospital, where my cousin SA worked, to find prescription blanks to write scripts on. I came down a set of stairs, opened the door and there she was. Oh shit, here I was with a suit and tie and in need of a quick excuse for what I was doing in one of the wings where I shouldn't have been. We exchanged hellos, and she asked, what are you doing here? Not meaning in the ward but at the hospital. I said a friend of mine needed a ride home and asked her to direct me to the ER where I could find him. Fuck! Talk about uncomfortable for me. I didn't find any prescription pads.

—"old and ready to retire"—

Doctor shopping is a term used for going to several doctors to find the ones that will write the prescriptions for the drugs you want. In the beginning, when I was trying to obtain Percocet, I'd go to *Urologists* for my fake scrotum problem.

One day, I found an MD in the phone book under *General Practitioners*. (I'd also look under *Family Medicine*, or if I was looking for cough syrup, I could use *ENT*—Ears Nose and Throat.) Well, here I was hoping to get Hycodan syrup, so I went to an MD on C. Street directly across from the hospital. I went into the waiting room, and one other person was there waiting. I looked around the room, and it had ancient everything, old pictures on the wall, an old fish tank with water but no fish in it. So, after the person before me came out, the doctor called me into an ancient examination room. No office furniture, no desk, just an examination table, and some really cool old medical equipment, like a full human skeleton model hanging by a wire from a hook. The doctor had me sit on the table and took some information from me, name, birthday, and why I was there.

These old doctors didn't want your address or phone number, they only wanted cash at the time of the visit. No billing, no nurse, and no secretary, just you and the doc and your money. So, to get the Hycodan, I needed to have a *non-productive cough*, meaning no phlegm and no congestion, just a dry hacking cough. Hopefully, the doctor wouldn't find the cause, since that would entail X-rays and all kinds of other unnecessary time-wasting things. He had me breathe to listen to my heart and lungs, then had me lie on my back. He had this gadget in his hand and a rubber tube in his mouth. He took a needle and pricked my fingertip, then took the glass tube that looked like an old eyedropper without the rubber bulb, where the rubber tube was connected. Then he put the glass eyedropper over the drop of blood from my fingertip and sucked the blood up into the glass tube through the rubber hose in his mouth. Then he put the blood on a glass microscope slide to examine the blood under the microscope on the shelf. Now I'd been there for well over an hour, between waiting and the examination. And he wasn't even close to being finished! Next, he walked behind me, pulled up his stool, sat down, and started to massage my temples and sinus passages over and under my eyes.

Now I was fine when I went in there, but by the time I sat up I was dizzy and my sinuses were clogged up and I couldn't breathe through my nose. The doctor had loosened up phlegm that I didn't even know I had. I have to say, he may have been old and ready to retire, which he did that year, but he was a very knowledgeable doctor. I got my cough syrup—a 4 oz bottle with no refills.

I went back a few times, but it was too much bullshit for too little medication.

—"one of a kind"—

There was a doctor on B. Ave in N. H., who was obviously near retirement. I think he felt that he had nothing to lose because the most the state could do to him was suspend his Schedule II narcotic privileges for a while. That's usually what the DCP does when a doctor or pharmacist abuses their privileges (meaning, prescribing too many narcotics unnecessarily). This doctor would only take cash, no medical insurance, no money orders, no personal checks, no credit cards, just good old cash money. The way he ran his practice was one of a kind that I had never seen before. First, you'd have to ring the doorbell, which was a buzzer. Second, you'd take a number off the hook on the wall. The numbers were on blocks of wood about 2 x 2 x ¼ inch thick. I was told that the numbers were so people wouldn't fight in the waiting room to see him first. He was a hilarious dude, not comic funny but strange funny. At any point, he might come out into the waiting room and say that's it for today and walk whoever was waiting to the door and lock it behind you. I was there when he pulled that shit one day.

After you took your number off the hook, you'd eventually be called in. The doctor never got out of his chair. He would have the previous patient leave the door open so he could yell NEXT. When you walked into his office, he would take the wooden block and check the number. He always had a cigarette in his mouth and his stethoscope around his neck. You'd sit down across from him at the desk, and he'd say what do you want? No what's wrong, no exam, just what do you want. LOL. Fucked up, huh? Anyway, I'd tell him, in my case, Percodan. He'd take out a crumpled-up prescription paper, not a full prescription pad, just loose scripts, and he'd write what I asked for. He would ask how many. If I said 40, he'd say 30, no bantering or argument. Kind of like the soup Nazi on *Seinfeld*. Once he was finished writing the prescription, he would reach across the desk, and you'd hand him the money. He would never hand you the prescription first. Once he had the money in his hand, he'd give you the prescription. Cigarette still in his mouth. If you changed your mind on what drugs you wanted, he'd toss the script he had just written in the trash, not even tear it up.

This doctor was a real piece of work. He would only be open Tuesday, Thursday, and Friday from 2 P.M. to 4 P.M. No phone number, no appointments, just a quick drug deal. As I said, he was coming to the end of his career in medicine. This was in 1979 or '80, and he was gone a year or two later.

There was another doctor on W. Ave in North H., and he was another old man that wanted to leave the medical profession with some pocket money. He would only prescribe drugs to certain girls. How he went about it was the girls needed to wear a dress, and he would sit next to them and just rub their leg. I asked a girl I knew that was seeing this doctor if he grabbed her pussy or wanted any sexual favors, but she said no that he just wanted to rub her leg!

Those kinds of doctors are still around, believe me. I just remained quiet for a while. I haven't kept that company for years now. They catered to doctor shoppers and girls who were drug addicts.

—"to be clean"—

I've made the difficult decision to get off of the Oxycodone. I started two days ago*. Going through a lot of depression, racing thoughts, fear. But it's something that I need to do, to be happy once again. Addiction consumes all of my life and leaves me with no life at all. I am already having a hard time sleeping for more than two hours at a time. I wake up drenched in sweat, then I'm ice cold even when I'm wrapped up in blankets. Last night I had a dream about being in a Methadone clinic. It's the second time I've dreamed of being back at the clinic, and in the dream, I am given the Methadone in two take-home bottles, but I wake up before I even leave the clinic. I wake up and begin to cry. I don't want to be on that death sentence taking that poison ever again. So, the way I'm going about this self-withdrawal is 5 mg every other day. Even at such a low dose, my mind and body don't want to give up the opioids. I know what it's like to be clean, and it's so much more enjoyable. But even with that knowledge, for some reason, my brain just refuses to let go.

*March 31, 2017—from a text message to the editor.

—"my entire body was on fire"—

While writing my story, I honestly forgot how opioid addiction can take hold of my life, my better judgment. I forgot how addictive Oxycodone is. I believed that all that I've been telling you was in the past. And that you, the reader, could only relate to the craziness by seeing me as a bystander. But after 13 years of being clean, I had to have surgery. I became addicted again. While telling you that I was taking prescribed Oxycodone makes it sound OK, well, it's not. And as all addicts do, I convinced myself of the lie because I didn't want to believe that I had become re-addicted to this very dangerous drug. It was much easier to deal with this time because I didn't have to fight so hard and so long to obtain the drug. I had a prescription!

During the times that I was forging prescriptions and doctor shopping, the DCP (Department of Consumer Protection) was trying to do what they were finally able to achieve only in 2017. I have been trying to stop using these pills going on two years now—to no avail. It took another frightening turn when my addiction took an unexpected path. I was running short on my prescribed meds, the Oxycodone. Before I became too sick to be able to do anything about it, I went to the city hospital emergency room. I needed enough pills to make it to my next doctor's appointment, which was a week away. In the ER, I found out that I have another bulging disk in my neck and have to go for an MRI. I also learned that the government now has a narcotics registry so that whenever I obtain a narcotic drug by prescription, it will automatically show up in the database. Of course, I made the hospital aware of my going to a pain clinic. That automatically put a stop to getting a prescription for any more narcotic pain medication.

I can't believe how I could have fallen into this state of addiction again. After everything it has done to my family and me. I am ashamed. Of myself and of what I have done. Even though I was not trying to get on pills again. I was so anti-opioid before my surgery that I refused to take the prescriptions that were written for me for other severe pain, for fear of becoming re-addicted. But because of the pain level I was experiencing with the new neck problem, I gave in to retaking them. Now it's been almost two years of being back on Oxycodone. I have been trying to get off the pills, and I now realize how difficult it is, how quickly we can forget the misery and pain we once experienced.

Well, here I am again, the first full day without *any* Oxycodone. I was bouncing all over my bed and haven't slept in 48 hours. This time I experienced not only legs and arms twitching, but my entire body was on fire.

I walked away from ten years of Methadone maintenance once I got down to 10 mg, and *that* was painful. When I was put in jail, I had to go cold turkey, from approximately 200 mg a day—that, plus 3 mg of Xanax—to zero. That experience was why I was never going to do narcotics again. How 13 years dulled my memory! I don't know if it's my age that is making it so difficult or what, but I can't believe I'm here again. I don't want to go on any other detox drugs or therapy. I need to remember that I was clean for 13 years and felt so good, and had no worries about the monster of being an addict hanging over my head.

I'm down from 70 mg a day to 15 mg a day and just about done. And I have learned what all the experts and past addicts, and even I know—I can't ever again take or do whatever I've once become addicted to, or I will always fall headfirst, back into the dark pit. No longer will I be able to play or be a weekend junkie. It's all or nothing. Because it's a *progressive disease*, this addict, or any addict, will soon surpass his previous addiction quantity of drugs. Or worse.

I *will* be clean, and I *will* be afraid of these drugs. And I will never think that I have the power to dictate to the drugs and not them to me. The drugs will always win.

—"nothing but a blur"—

When I started doing opioids, 1979-1980, these drugs were prescribed regularly for moderate to severe pain. Drugs such as Demerol, Percodan, Tylox, and Percocet became everyday meds, but you rarely would see Dilaudid prescribed. It would only be for cancer patients or others with severe pain.

By the late '80s, doctors were asked by the state DCP to slow down prescribing the Oxycodone family of pain meds. And by the early '90s, when I was asked by the state to work with the local ABC news affiliate, things were coming to a head. All-out war was being waged against the opioid drugs. But the owners of Percocet and Percodan weren't going down easy, as they were making huge sums by just putting their name on the #1 selling opioid pain medication in my state, if not the entire country. Half-way through the six-part series that I was in, the TV station received a telephone call from the manufacturer. I don't know, but I'm sure it was their representative and not their legal team.

The investigating reporter told me the company VP was going to fly up to refute the claims that I had made about the addictiveness of their drug. The company was less than pleased with my statement. Now I don't scare easily or get intimidated by many people. But this worried me because a drug user like me would be nothing to them for me to not exist anymore, not if the decision comes to my life or millions of dollars. I have never been threatened nor even approached by anyone from any company. But I took the precaution of calling the state DCP head agent at the time. It was probably just my paranoia. As it turned out, the vice president of the manufacturer never did show up at the TV station.

Things began to slow down with the prescribing of opioids until Purdue Pharma introduced OxyContin (Oxycodone) to the marketplace. Overnight the opioid problem was in full swing, and opioids were everywhere. I began to forge prescriptions for the 40 mg and 80 mg pills and made a lot of money for about two years. I would sell the majority of the pills while only taking a couple of them a day. I was well into being addicted to OxyContin. I was also on Methadone. And after 10 years of being on that poison, I began getting the Duragesic (Fentanyl) 100 mcg patches prescribed to me by pain specialists. I got so Fentanyl dependent that I wore a patch once a day. Supposed to last 3 days. I even cut the corner of the patch and put drops of the Fentanyl under my tongue, all while wearing a new Duragesic patch. I consumed so many of these patches that I had to sell my Harley Davidson to pay for them. I had bought the Harley a year earlier for $15,000 cash. Only 1,000 miles later, I sold it for $10,000 cash. Within a few weeks, I had spent all that money on Duragesic patches. They were $500 for a box of ten 100 mcg patches. Ten thousand dollars didn't last long. At the time, I also had stopped selling OxyContin and Percocet.

I'm trying to remember exactly when each of these events occurred. Life was nothing but a blur while on Fentanyl. I'd say it had to be 8 months before I went to prison for a lifetime of being arrested. Sentenced to 4 years for the sale of seven Xanax pills.

When I was being booked to go into prison, I had a Duragesic patch in my mouth. The About the Author photo shows how I looked at the time.

I had never been arrested for any kind of drug sales before in my life. With all the money I made in my 20+ years, and thousands of pills sold, it took only 7 Xanax pills to end all of the destructive madness for the people whose lives I helped destroy, and for me. Like my son and mother said to me, if I hadn't been arrested and put in prison, I'd be dead. And they both told me to use the time in prison to better myself and become healthy again. If not for my family, I would have given up and not cared about what happened to me at the time. I was at a place where I welcomed death as I would lay there in prison barely alive, in health and in spirit. I was literally at death's door. I have so much to be thankful for now in my life, and it's not the end of my story, because I need to get back to the good life of being clean.

Now, after a year and a half of chronic pain following my neck surgery, I have yet to get off Oxycodone. And I will. Because I prefer drug-free life over every morning's hangover with no money, no job. It is decision time: to live miserably or happy again. It's not a close call. I have loved being drug-free, and springing out of bed in the morning with a new day to take head-on. And enjoy.

—"an intelligent addict"—

Consistency. Consistency was the reason that I turned to prescription drugs. Purity. Purity was another reason. I got tired of buying street drugs and getting high and then returning to purchase the same drug from the same person and not getting the same results. The variation in street drugs sucks. If I'm going to spend my hard-earned money on something, I expect to get the same product. But it doesn't work that way in the street drug business. That was how I ended up taking only prescription drugs. The opioids. If I didn't get the same reaction each time from the prescription drugs, I knew it was because of me, not the seller. That I hadn't eaten, and my body didn't have the energy to burn. When I was speeding, I noticed that I would fall into a depressed state, but if I ate some food, it would kick in the high or the euphoric feeling again. Trying to get the best bang for my buck, I became much more addicted because of the reasons I chose to do them over the street drugs. They were much better in purity, consistency, always delivering what I expected. Still, I didn't expect to become addicted! That's why I insist that the difference between street Heroin and prescription Oxycodone is like night and day. And, you can stop one much more easily than the other.

If you were able to get pure Heroin, the comparison wouldn't even be close, the Heroin would be much more potent than Oxycodone. But if you are lucky, you are only going to find between 3% and 5% Heroin. It has been claimed that 8% purity in the strength of street Heroin was killing people. And now who knows what you are getting when you buy Heroin; it's mostly garbage, with a little Fentanyl added. And people are dying from that.

It's consistency, and the longer half-life of an opioid, that creates addiction. When I witnessed Heroin addicts quit the drug, they would only experience withdrawals for 3 days. But for a person addicted to pharmaceutical drugs like Oxycodone, the withdrawals easily last 30 days. My psychiatrist, who was a chemical dependency expert, told me that it could take me up to 18 months to get a sleeping pattern down. Very discouraging. Thinking that I was being slick or an intelligent addict, which was careless, I became more addicted. What it all comes down to is that prescription drugs are not something that you want to abuse.

It starts out all fun and games and ends up a life and death situation.

—"old enough for me"—

I used to forge prescriptions for 4 mg tablets of Dilaudid. At the time, this was the strongest the manufacturer made. Now they also make 8 mg, but back in the '80s and '90s, when I was getting them, they only had 2 and 4 mg tablets. So, of course, I would write for the higher dose. At first, I sold them for $25 a pill.

About 1998, I was talking to a buddy of mine that lived in Daytona Beach. The same guy I did LSD with for the first time (and first got arrested with, too). At the time, junkies in Florida weren't able to get Heroin, and would pay good money for Dilaudid, like up to $50 a pill. For one lousy pill! So, I told my buddy in Daytona that if he could sell enough of the pills, I'd fly down and give them to him for $35 a pill. By the time I was ready to go down there, I had 500 pills of Dilaudid to bring with me. We made a date that I'd be down to Daytona Beach. He needed to have the money ready. I didn't want to be stuck carrying pills around Florida and definitely didn't want them on me when I flew home. Now 500 x $50 is $25,000. I would give him $5,000 to sell them in one shot, to one person. Just to have company, I asked another friend of mine if he'd like to go with me to Florida for a week and stay on the beach in a hotel.

My wife—who in only a month or two would be my ex-wife—drove us to the airport, and me and my friend flew to Daytona Beach. We got there, and I couldn't get hold of my Florida buddy until late that night. I said, when are we going to meet the guy with the money? Oh, he answered, I'm sorry, but he was arrested 2 days ago. I said, why didn't you call and tell me? He said, well, I thought that we'd hang out for a week and party. Party? I just wasted $3,000 on a flight and hotel room for a week. I wasn't in no mood to hang out and party. I was fucking pissed off because instead of making $20,000, I was in the hole for $3,000 already. I had 500 pills of Dilaudid in the hotel safe in the room and about $1,000 on me, to eat, play, etc.

So, me and the guy I flew down with went to a strip joint right off the main drag. Now I always had the gift of gab with strippers, and especially when I had drugs on me. I looked 10 times more handsome to the girls, but didn't we all? LOL. I met a pretty young girl from Maine who was dancing, and she had a best friend who was also dancing that night. They were both addicted to ketamine or KAT, something I had never done. It sounded like it was actually powdered Angel Dust or Wet, as they call it now. I still have pictures of us all together in the hotel room and eating at Denny's. Anyway, I asked them to come back to the hotel with us because by then, my friend was hitting it off with my stripper's blonde partner. And instead of giving my stripper money while she was dancing, I was giving her Dilaudid. Which she loved because of how much money she could sell them for in Daytona. Instead of dollar bills, I'd put pills in her G-string. The two girls and my friend were smoking pot that my Daytona buddy gave me, in case we ran into some girls. These girls were beautiful, in their late teens or maybe early 20s. I didn't ask, didn't care. If they were able to strip legally, that was old enough for me.

After the second day going into the strip joint in Daytona, that night with the girls back at the hotel room, they told me that the owner didn't want me back there because I was selling them drugs. I had the same problem at a strip joint back home.

That whole trip was a waste of time, money, and pills. Just another couple of days in the drug business. A world that I no longer miss. Not one bit.

—"under surveillance"—

During all the years of addiction, my wife was addicted too. But only close friends knew. I would never let the law know. In 1982 and '84, I begged her to let me go into rehab, and when I came out, she would go in. But she refused. So, I just kept doing what I had to. She would steal my pills, and I would know because I'd keep them counted. She would break into my briefcase by fiddling with the combinations, and take the pills. We'd always argue, and it put a lot of stress on everybody. Very tiring. Lots of anxiety.

It got to the point where I would get very dizzy. I'd have to crawl to the bathroom, crawl to the couch. I couldn't stand up. I didn't know what it was; I thought it was a brain tumor. The anxiety and depression were out of control. Eventually, my mother-in-law told me she believed it was anxiety. She gave me the name of the psychiatrist she was seeing. I went there and was told it was indeed anxiety. This was *after* I went to neurologists, orthopedic doctors, and ear, nose, and throat doctors. I had thought perhaps I had a middle ear problem.

The psychiatrist put me on a few things that didn't work. He told me to get off the Percocet before he'd give me anything else. I told him I was clean, and he put me on Zoloft and Xanax. I held onto the Xanax for a week, too scared to take them. Finally, it was Christmas, and my wife and son were headed out to visit relatives. I had to do something, so I took half a Xanax, and, boom! Anxiety gone. I said I'd go with them and my wife almost fell over. I spent about an hour but ended up feeling dizzy and nervous again. I went home, took another one, and went back to the family.

The depression was still there. Every night I would go out to get more drugs, and cry, wishing I was at home with my son, playing with his Matchbox cars. Just being home with my family. But I couldn't, I still had a full-time job. Not only were we addicted, but I also couldn't hold a regular job because I always needed the pills. Plus, I had to sell the pills to live. Terrible way to live.

I kept getting arrested. Lawyer bills added up, $3000 here, $1000 there. By then, the DCP picked up on me. I was arrested in W., and the detective that interrogated me called me a few days afterward and told me they wanted to talk to me. They knew about the pharmacist I was buying drugs from because they had the pharmacy under surveillance. I did not want to go to jail. Yes, I had a problem, my wife had a problem, and, I had a son. I just couldn't disappear for a year. It was the hardest thing I ever had to do.

When I was summoned to the DCP in the state capital, the drug control unit got me to sit down and talk with them. They asked me—or told me? I don't remember—if I would be willing to help the Ivy League college hospital tighten their security. To prevent any more prescription pads from being stolen. They didn't realize that I was the only one who was stealing those scripts. Or maybe they did but wouldn't say. They also asked me if I was willing to meet with the local ABC TV news station. And last but not least, to meet with some detectives… just to talk. I said yes to all three requests.

A few days had gone by when I got a call from the college police. We met at the hospital, and I walked two detectives around, one of them a young woman. I explained to them that if they told the doctors and nurses to just leave the cabinet drawers open and not locked, the thieves wouldn't think anything worth taking was in them. After walking through the hospital and pointing out several things, we got to the end of the tour. I heard this loud click, so I looked at the male detective and said, your tape recorder just turned off. He turned red from embarrassment and reached into his pocket and pulled out the recorder and turned it completely off.

—"for the sake of my art"—

The second call came from the TV news station, an investigative reporter on the phone asking me for an interview, so I agreed. All of these favors would be reported to the prosecutor and the lawyers who wanted me locked up.

We set up a date, and I went to the news station in N. H., and the reporter wanted me to speak with him on camera. I told him not happening. I didn't tell him that I was still actively forging scripts. And to put my face with my red hair and overweight ass on TV would result in all of the state police force converging on the station to arrest me. Nope, not happening. We came to an agreement to talk with my face blacked out.

The reporter wanted me to show how I got the R paper—the prescription paper or scripts. He and a photographer with an oversized VHS camcorder accompanied me to the local public hospital. I was not dressed up in my customary suit and tie. I grabbed my pry bar and hid it under the winter coat I was wearing. I showed them where to park and took the pry bar. Because I was definitely not going to waste my time without seizing some script paper. The reporter freaked out and asked what was I doing with the pry bar? I told him that if he wanted to see how it was done, I was going to have to show him. He got all nervous and said we couldn't be committing any crimes while we did this. So, I put the pry bar under the front seat of the van we were in and laughed at him. Now the photographer started to laugh at the reporter. I said, everyone wants to be a criminal without doing the crime. LOL.

We got into the hospital. The photographer had his camcorder in a gym type bag with matching webbing so that the camera could be used incognito. I started to look for prescription pads, and the reporter was sweating from nervous anxiety. He had had enough and wanted to go home and lay down in a fetal position and suck his thumb. LOL. Actually, we went back to the studio where he interviewed me.

The next day the reporter wanted me to show him how I doctor-shopped. I had made an appointment the day before the visit. They picked me up, and as we were driving to the doctor's office, they asked how the photographer was going to be in the room with me. I said, what do you mean in the examination room with me? He said that they needed to photograph how I did it. Now I was pretty much fucking disgusted with this clown. Still, for the sake of my art, I agreed and told the cameraman that I was going to introduce him as my brother-in-law. This was the first time I'd ever seen this doctor, and it was already a fucking disaster. I was called into the exam room with this 6-foot 5-inch black man behind me. What the fuck, it doesn't work like this. LOL. The doctor asked me what the matter was, so I told him that my balls were injured and so he took hold and said, turn your head and cough.

I got a prescription for Percocet. Now I had planned on having it filled. But the reporter said oh no we can't because we obtained it illegally and started in with his crying bullshit again, so I relented and let him have the script. If I had done it without the state being involved, fat chance that he would have gotten my script. LOL. But I had to behave and just get the shit done with.

The TV piece I did for them, a 6-part series, was used for sweeps week—for ratings. Now me and my son and wife had moved in with my parents, and they watched that news channel at 6 P.M. when the special would air. I was so embarrassed and ashamed of myself that I didn't want to face them. Plus, this was showing all week with the 6th episode slipped in somewhere. Even though my face was blacked out, the camera still showed the rings that were on my fingers. I had two or three nice diamond rings on. And my voice and the way that I spoke was a dead giveaway to anyone that knew me. The very first night that it aired, I got a phone call from a buddy who was one of the guys that I started with, and as soon as I said hello, he said, "Hey, Woody!" so I knew who it was. He said, what the fuck, man. I asked him how did you know it was me? He said, the gold rings. LOL

— "all of these favors"—

The hardest and most demeaning thing that the state asked me to do for them was, to expect a call from the statewide narcotics task force. A few days after that, I received a call from a guy who asked me to meet him at the back of a nearby diner, so I said OK. Now I didn't know if I was going to be blackmailed or what to expect. I needed some kind of insurance because all of these favors I was doing just to have a good word put into the local superior court was becoming really fucking old. I wasn't happy about being so involved with the enemy of my prescription forgery business.

On the other hand, I thought that they could be a great help to me, not only then but in the future. I turned out to be right! Anyway, I needed to have some insurance just in case. In case of what and who would I turn to even if they were going to blackmail me. I wasn't in any position to be holding anything over anyone's head. My back was up against the wall, and I had the most important thing in my life to worry about, and that was my family who needed me and, I thought, couldn't live without me.

Sometimes I wonder if I put too much importance on my role as a husband and father.

Anyway, I drove down the street to Radio Shack. I bought a small tape recorder and a tiny microphone to record my conversation with the statewide narcotics agents. Back in the mid to late '80s, nothing was miniaturized like they are now. It was a voice-activated recorder.

The day came to meet with the agents. I went there and made sure that I arrived before anyone else, so I could scope out who, where, why, and when. Eventually, the agents pulled up. I had told them what I would be driving, as if they didn't know already. They pulled up next to me, and I got into the back seat of their car. The driver introduced himself and was in the process of introducing the guy in the passenger seat when I said, how are you doing, Mr. Jones. Not his real name, but for the story, Jones will be fine. He said to the driver, he knows who I am. They told me that they wanted me to be a rat, an informant for them, and explained how it was to be done. I thought it would be like just telling them some names, and we'd be all set. Well, they had different plans and their own ways of doing the job.

First of all, I didn't like the state agent that I already knew. Second, they wanted me to go around my home town—where I was trusted and knew everyone in it! I grew up in that town! They wanted me to go into the bars and clubs and introduce a cop, or cops, to people who were selling drugs, cocaine, and whatever else we could buy? In fact, I never hung around the bar scene. I was a married man and father, and I already wasn't home enough because of doing scripts. I offered up another scenario, but that wasn't going to work for them. In the end, I was introduced to another cop from a nearby town. I began to go around the bars and clubs in that town, presenting him as a friend of the family.

During the time I worked for these guys, I continued to get arrested in towns all around the state. And kept piling up court dates. They offered to help me with each court case in each town.

As far as the tape recorder goes, I never needed it. A few years afterward, I told the agent, now my buddy, that I had taped the conversation. He just laughed and said that he'd been taped by better people than me. LOL.

During all this time nobody ever suspected that my wife was an addict. 'cause that's how I wanted it to be. Once people found out, they were in shock. Some never believed that she was. But that's OK.

—"everyone did it"—

The cop that I knew from my home town became a good friend, and I grew to have a lot of respect for him. Still do. He's one of the most honest cops I know. I found out that he was so good at his job working undercover that he worked with the statewide narcotics task force for over ten years. The task force usually employed local cops for no more than a year. These cops were on loan from each town and had their duties in that particular town. But this guy was so good that the state wanted him forever.

So good, in fact, that the state gave him Corvettes, beautiful custom Harleys, and Cadillacs. He was the cream of the crop when it came to undercover work. I was worried that he wouldn't have the same pull in the courts of other towns as he did in the local court. Well, in some of them anyway, he wielded even more power and influence. In some of my court cases, I'd go in to talk to the head prosecutor, and they would hold my court folder over the trash can in their office and just drop it in and tell me not to come back to their town again. It seemed like they all either owed my buddy or had tremendous respect for him, or both. While I was getting arrested all around my home state, 99% of the police departments would know my buddy. And when I would mention his name, they would make a phone call, and I would be released without bond and with only a signature.

I don't know if it was such a good thing for me to have him as a connection and as a good friend. Or actually a bad thing.

By the way, those beautiful vehicles were just to use for his job, even though he drove them as if they were his.

That's how I was able to stay out of jail for so long, even though I would joke with him about how he would know every time I sold a single pill. I'd tell him to just make it easy for me and tell me only the names of the people who *didn't* work for him because it became clear that a lot more people in my town were in his pocket than just me. LOL.

Whenever the people who I ratted on were able to figure out who set them up, I would just tell them that I did it. And that if they had a problem with me, do something now, because I'm going to be ending the informant thing and going home. That none of it was personal, just business. I think that threw them for a loop because I never hid it, even though it destroyed my credibility. I did manage to keep a little dignity for telling them that I was the one. Still, each time one of my workers got busted, I would send them to my buddy, and they too would end up working for the statewide narcotics task force and wouldn't go to jail. But some of them wouldn't be as honest as I was, or as crazy as I was, and they would try to keep it a well-hidden secret. Few would ever admit that they were snitching, but everyone did it for their own personal reasons. Mine was so I could provide for my family. Once they were no longer in need of me to provide for them, I stopped fighting and just let the state put me away in prison. Which was an easier decision to make instead of completely destroying my name and dignity.

—"piss for probation"—

I had to tell my probation officer that I was busted again since he expected to see me. Every time I saw my probation officer, he took a urine sample. I've been giving urine to the probation department or the Methadone clinics my whole life, 30 years of giving up urine. When I had to piss for probation, if I had dirty urine, I was going to jail for violating. So right from the start, I had to come up with a way to give clean urines that were at body temperature.

The people who take the urine watch you so you can't give them someone else's urine from a different bottle. There is a strip on the container you are given for temperature readings so that you can't give someone else's urine. I had a soft plastic bottle from a radio control airplane with some flesh-colored rubber fuel line for the airplane fuel system. I made a hole in the top of the screw cap and attached a stem onto it, so I could attach the rubber hose. I put the bottle under my armpit, held in place with a rubber band, and ran the tube down my arm. I always wore a long-sleeved shirt. The hose ran under my watch band into the palm of my hand. I would use a Lite-Brite peg from the game as a plug or stopper. When I gave the urine, I would just squeeze my arm to my body and fill their bottle.

Now, here's the trick: I would have my young son pee in a cup and tell him that it was for his pediatrician to make sure that he was healthy. Sad. But that's how I had clean urines all the time.

My probation officer questioned me about this latest arrest. I told him what had happened, and he pulled out a picture of me in my Halloween get-up, the cervical collar, and the red food coloring as blood. He got a kick out of it. He got a clean urine sample, and I was free to leave.

The best part of being arrested in B. was the big shot detective. He was an asshole with a real attitude. He told me that HE was the statewide narcotics task force. Yup, he thought he was such a fucking big shot. For my second court date in D., my buddy with the statewide narcotics task force—the agent that actually had power—told me to talk to Inspector So-and-so, the court inspector up there. I went in and sat in the courtroom and looked up at the judge who was sitting there. It turned out to be the same judge who had just given me three years of probation in N. H. superior court! What the fuck were the chances of that? Judges move around from court to court after a few months, or a year or so. I couldn't believe it. I slumped down into the seat so as not to be seen by him, even though I had red hair and weighed 250 pounds at the time, and where would I hide? Ain't happening. I got called out of the courtroom by the guy who my buddy told me to talk to, the Inspector mentioned earlier. We walked into his office. He had my folder in his hand and said, don't come back, and dropped the folder into the trash can. I thanked him, and he said, thank your friend from B., and I left. I will always remember that cocky detective who said that he was such a big shot. My buddy had more pull in his courthouse than he did. That's how much power my hometown buddy had … throughout the whole state.

—"with these regrets"—

The most significant part of this life that I've led is all the regrets. My life is full of them. My biggest regrets are the pain and suffering I've inflicted upon my family. I love them all so much, and I've hurt them equally as much. My son, he's seen half the man who I truly am because of my drug addiction. I can't make up for the time I've squandered away. I can only hope that he doesn't choose to make the same mistakes and then have the same regrets as I do. Like my parents, and all parents, I want only the very best and the greatest happiness for my child.

My mother was always by my side, picking me up every time I fell down, no matter what. No ex-wife, no ex-girlfriend, and no buddies were there to send me money or visit or write to me while I was in prison. Only my family was there for me. My poor son only came to visit me twice in those 30 months of prison. That shows me how much it hurt him to see me in that predicament. My younger brother came up from Florida and took time out of his only vacation in years to come to see me behind bars. My sister came to visit a couple of times and cried when she saw me. My father wanted so badly to see me but couldn't because the prison wasn't wheelchair accessible. And within a month of my incarceration, he passed away. I never got to hold him and tell him that I loved him before he died. But I did tell him my whole life. I have always kissed all of my family members hello and goodbye my entire life because I love them. You just never know when or if you're going to see them again. But my son was at my father's side when he passed away, so I know that he was representing me. My dad had to have known that.

I will live with these regrets for the rest of my life. Those who know me know I have a good heart and am there for them if they need me. It's the drugs and only the drugs that have hindered me my entire life, and diminished my potential. And shattered my dreams, as well as my needs and every other aspect of my being.

I can't stress enough how lousy chemical abuse can be to life and soul, including for all of those who love you. It isn't just the addict who is hurt by drugs, but everyone in your life. Sorry doesn't cut it after a while, and regrets don't help heal the people that you've hurt.

I do wish my dad could see the real me and not the drug-high me. I know that he'd be proud of me even though my loved ones say that he knows and understands. It's just not the same as his saying that to me in person. We can never go back, but like a great white shark, to live, we must keep moving forward, or die. We can only learn and grow by our mistakes, hopefully, and continue to grow and move forward.

—"intervention"—

In 1982 I had enough sense to know that me and my wife had a drug problem with the Percodan, Percocet, and Tylox. All three drugs contain the same opioid, Oxycodone. We'd been taking them every day for a little over a year, and I was desperate to quit, so I told my wife that I would get enough pills for her so that I could go into a 30-day detox, and when I got out, she could go in. The reasoning behind that was so one of us would be there to take care of our son. Well, she cried and was frightened of the idea but didn't want me to go and get clean. So no detox.

In 1984 and even further into our addiction, my mom, dad, sister, and younger brother held an intervention for me. Without any knowledge of what was about to happen, I went to my parents' house, and my sister drove in right behind me, blocking my car from leaving. They told me that I needed help with drugs. My parents offered to watch our son while we (me and my wife) got help. At that time, they actually didn't know that my wife had a drug problem. It was only as we talked that they found out about the both of us. That's when they said we both should go get help, and they would take care of our son. I told them that I was scared to go and my dad said, "Don't you think that I was scared when I was in the concentration camp?" and he began to cry. What was I going to say to that? Not a thing except "I know Dad." I had never seen my dad cry before, and I was the one who caused it. I told them that I would talk it over with my wife.

I told her what our options were, and she got angry at my family for, as she put it, sticking their noses into our business. Pretty cold of her to feel like that when all they wanted to do was help us. So twice in two years, I asked and pleaded with her to allow us to get off the drugs. Both times she refused. But once she was clean, she told me I should have done what I needed to do. Wow, what a fucking bitch. I truly hated her guts with all of my heart and soul at that moment.

My ex-wife was baptized at the same church we both attended, even though she was still on Methadone. The church knew that we both were in the Methadone program. Yet, when she was being baptized, I asked the church why she was ready for baptism and not I, even though we were at the same places in all aspects of the religion, that being the bible studies, the church attendance, everything. Well, they felt that she was ready and that I wasn't. Yeah, she had tits and I didn't. That's the only difference that I could see.

Years later, once she had got clean, and off Methadone before I was, she was acting holier than me. Now that she was excelling in life and I was lagging behind, I said to her one day that I wished that she had allowed me to have gone into the 30-day detox those years ago. Her reply was, you should have. Really? I should have? Wow, I guess she didn't remember the resistance she put up and the guilt she made me feel.

This is just some of the nitty-gritty of the things that we addicts go through and feel. I know you already know this, I'm just afraid of the pain of reliving this being lost, being for nothing.

—"grateful"—

I have been such a fuckup, ruining my life for good jobs and rights like hunting or owning a firearm. I am grateful that my beautiful son has never been arrested or ever had a fistfight. He has turned out to be a wonderful and gentle man. He is much more intelligent than I. He always thinks before acting, never jumps to conclusions, or reacts to emotions. He knows how to utilize the English language correctly, he has beautiful handwriting. He is what every parent dreams of for a child. I don't know how, except that he must have seen how I lived my life and did the complete opposite. He is my pride and joy and makes me feel like my life hasn't been a total waste of time. And my parents, thank God for them, they have always shown me love even when it must have been impossible to love me. My whole family has never wavered in their love for me, and that keeps me in line. Otherwise, I would give up.

—"just to survive"—

When I was sent to prison, it was my only real vacation. I was able to read a lot of books, play chess, exercise, and even sleep some of the time. Sleeping's hard to do, what with all the assholes making noise and flushing toilets 24/7. I can only offer this advice: don't ever start doing drugs. Life is hard and complicated enough without a ten-ton weight on your back. I had no time to be a father or husband. Whenever I was home, while on drugs, I suffered from such severe anxiety and depression that I could barely *stand up* because of severe dizziness from the stress. I had to do almost everything lying down. Like while playing with my son, whether Legos or Matchbox cars, or while watching movies. Even after I was prescribed Xanax, I was still a mental wreck. Once I became an addict, I never did drugs to get really high, but just to maintain and to not get sick. Hardly living, barely existing. The drugs were just to survive.

You must realize that I was very aware of the toll that all of this shitty nightmare was taking on my entire family. Not just my wife and son, but also my mother and father and sister and brother. On top of which my sister worked for the local police department. She's been there for 35 plus years, so it wasn't like I could keep it hidden from her. She couldn't or wouldn't tell our parents about me, probably because of the law, and not to make them worry about her fuck-up of a brother. Always was and still am.

Through it all, my family has always loved me. It would have been much easier for them not to.

—"being clean"—

Even with all the love and support we may get, drug addicts need to take responsibility for their own actions. A parent can only hold their child's hand for so long. We are responsible for our own lives and our decisions, good or bad. Life is hard, especially nowadays, much more than when I was young. Too many choices and too many outside influences. But lots of options can be a good thing also. Kids have so many choices and opportunities today; it just comes down to the choices that you make in your life. I tell friends who get high that life being clean is good. You absorb much more of everything, love, nature, food, and even pain and suffering. You're able to come to terms with your problems instead of rehashing them over and over again. They never get better when you're high because you're not mentally capable of putting them in their proper perspective. You carry them around with you forever. You don't grow intellectually.

I now figure that when I got out of prison, I was still 16 years old and had to grow up all over again.

I never liked the NA or AA programs because it seemed to me that I was just reliving the things that I wanted to distance myself from, grow away from. They reminded me of my failures over and over every week. I needed to work and be responsible for myself and keep moving forward like my proverbial shark, keep moving forward or die. Don't get me wrong, some people utilize the programs very well and benefit tremendously from them. Still, in every one of my program situations, I was forced by court order to attend. Not by my own free will. Ultimately, you do what you have to do to get better. Everybody is different and different things work for different people.

Rehabs don't work. It takes something in your life or actually your brain to be shocked into a different state of mind. Mine was prison, but I know a lot of people who were imprisoned much longer than I, came out and picked up right where they stopped, just like the girl in this story who died in her parents' bathtub. Most do die if they return to the drugs. I've tried to figure out why. I honestly believe that either your body or a higher power says no, I can't go through this again. Because most of the people who died that I knew didn't take more or even pick up where they left off when they had quit. It's the body or mind shutting down for its own protection, that's my thinking anyway.

—"another finely orchestrated and executed plan"—

Me and two guys—three stooges—had robbed a pharmacy, a case that went unsolved, at least by the state police major crime division. Seven months after the crime, I solved it for them. Out of guilt, I turned myself in for doing the job.

On one of the nights that we three guys weren't able to get a prescription filled, we decided to rob another local pharmacy. We didn't have any weapons, only a can of police mace that one of the kids had stolen from his brother who was a cop. We already had this particular pharmacy in mind, knowing that it had a front door and a back door.

We were waiting for the store to close. The plan was for all three of us to wait until the pharmacist and the cashier came out the back door and, right before they locked the door and activated the alarm, we would have them go back into the pharmacy and give us the drugs. We waited and waited, and waited some more. We knew that the store closed at 9 P.M., but the lights were still on, so we continued to wait. It got to be 9:45, and something clearly wasn't right. One of the guys went to the front door to see what the heck was going on. He came back and told us the pharmacy was closed. What? I said. It's closed. We all walked around to the front, and sure enough it was closed, locked up tight. Lights off. What happened, we asked each other, more than a little baffled. I guess they had gone out the front door, the light on at the back of the store was always on overnight.

Another finely orchestrated and executed plan. This is what drug addiction desperation can lead to.

—"her son was a junkie"—

I trained a so-called buddy of mine, by the name of Bobby, during my last two years of forging prescriptions. Now, most if not all of the people you do drugs with, or buy, sell drugs with or to, are just acquaintances. If they indeed are friends, it won't be for long once you sell drugs to them because then there emerges a client-supplier mentality. And the client or buyer ends up being resentful towards the drug seller. It's a natural human reaction, I guess. Everything having to do with drugs is temporary.

The people I would teach how to act and watch after while they were in the pharmacy... they were all drug addicts. They wouldn't have any money to purchase the prescription with. I not only provided the prescription papers, but wrote them, found the pharmacies, knew which ones were cool, used my car, and paid for them. Therefore, I wasn't going to split the pills 50:50. Not happening. So, I came up with a percentage system. For instance, if I wrote for 40 Percocet pills—the smallest amount I would write, considering the risk—I would give the person 15 pills, and I would keep 25. Sometimes, even giving them just 10 pills. Depending on how fed up I felt for doing absolutely all the work. On 60 pills, which was the standard quantity that I would write for, I would give them 20 and keep 40; on 80 pills, I would give them 25 and keep 55. Even if they supplied their own money, I still wasn't splitting the pills 50:50. Basically, I would discourage them from using their own money, because it was not in my best interest to do all the work and give up half the pills.

Now, because Bobby had such a high drug tolerance, he wanted more of the pills than I would usually provide. The only way for him to get more than half was by having stolen his mother's Medicaid card. That way, no cash had to be used in the transaction. Bobby told me to write his mother's name on the forged prescriptions that he would use. I felt that if he had no problems with using his own mother's name, birthday, address, phone number, and everything else, then so be it. This went on for a few months. Finally, the E. H. police department called his mother and notified her that her Medicaid card was being used to obtain narcotics with forged prescriptions. She knew that her son was a junkie. And that every day we were up to no good. She would even call me regularly to make sure her son wasn't getting too high. She would ask that I make sure he got home safely. Yeah, I'm a fucking babysitter, sweetheart, keep him home with you if he needs to be babysat. But I would be polite, and tell her that I'd make sure that he was OK.

The police wanted Bobby to come down to the station so they could take a mug shot of him. That way, they could bring his picture around to all the pharmacies in town. I told him to tell the police to either get a warrant or arrest him because that was bullshit. But he thought he was such a genius and went out and bought a fake beard from a nearby Halloween store. Well, he came over to my house to apply the dead rat to his face. It sure didn't look like a beard. I even told him it resembled a dead rat. Still, I couldn't convince him. Even my girlfriend couldn't believe that he was going to pass this nonsense off, especially with the police. LOL. Oh lord, he finally finished putting the monstrosity on his face. With all the tweaking and trying to get it to look right, he had the glue or makeup gum all over the beard's hair, and there were bald spots where he missed and then places where he had cut some off and put it in different spots. You get the picture. It was a fucking mess. I told him to just forget it and make them serve him a warrant. Anyway, he went to the police station with the dead rat glued to his face. After all that, every single pharmacy in E. H. identified Bobby as the culprit by the time a warrant came back from the court. LOL.

I had moved to my parents' house and shortly after that was arrested for helping that girl that I mentioned earlier when I stopped to help her out with the Xanax. So, I went to court in N. H., where my buddy Bobby had gone for the scripts that he was busted for while using his mother's insurance card on (my) forged prescriptions. Like anyone who has been arrested and has made a lot of money in the drug selling business, I couldn't afford an attorney. So, I applied for a public defender. The next court date I had, I went into the public defenders' office. One of the other lawyers told me that they couldn't defend me because of a conflict of interest. I said, what do you mean by conflict of interest? She asked me if I knew a Bobby so-and-so. I said, Yeah. She told me that he was blaming me for sending him into all the pharmacies that he was arrested at for obtaining drugs with a forged prescription. This, I'm sure, was told him by the police, so that he could get off of all the charges if he gave me up. Every cop in the state knew that it was me behind all of the forged prescriptions… in the entire state. And they wanted to put me away for a long time, but couldn't do it because of my connection with the chief state attorney's office through my friend from my home town. But Bobby also had done some favors for the same guy as I had, but he refused to help Bobby this time.

The public defender's office told me to find another attorney. But I had no money, so they assigned me a *special* public defender that the state had on retainer for such cases as mine. But wait till I tell you this crazy story about the *special* public defender that they gave me.

A few months before this court date, my girlfriend Kerry had gotten arrested in N. H. for armed robbery. My buddy from my home town had talked to her through me because he was interested in the woman (her mother) who she lived with before I met her. Her mother married this guy who was the head of the LK gang. She resided in F. H., and Kerry lived with this woman. When I met Kerry, I told her I didn't want anyone knowing my business and I didn't want to know her business, and left it at that. My police buddy had arranged for Kerry to get off with a few years of probation instead of jail time. But the lawyer that the state appointed for her was not allowing the deal to go through. That's what my buddy told me as he was coming out of the judge's chambers. She was going to be receiving 3 years in the women's prison. I was upset because of this motherfucker of a lawyer who, instead of helping her, stuck it to her. I sat down in the big federal court and waited for her to go before the judge and be sentenced. She came up from the holding cell, and we looked at each other, not really knowing what to expect because no matter what deals were made, the judge had the final say. I was waiting, and she went before the judge. Her lawyer did absolutely nothing to help her or offer any positive words in her defense. Kerry got 3 years. There goes another girl who I had feelings for, right out of my life. And her life, gone also. I was crying, and the lawyer came walking by, and I got up and told him that I was gonna fuck him up when we got outside. The sheriffs ran over to stop the argument. This lawyer was short, and I said, while the sheriffs had us separated, I'm going to smack you on the top of your head and make you even shorter.

Fast forward to my court appearance in the other court in N. H., superior court now, before I was scheduled for my first appearance for violating probation. I was locked up in North Ave. Jail. This place was so old that in what they called the Flats, they had cells where the doors were still closed manually by a massive arm at the end of the row of cells. This place was built in the 1800s. I was transported to the superior court and waited to see the lawyer I had been appointed by the public defenders' office (my "special" public defender). My so-called buddy, my trainee Bobby, told the court I was at fault for sending him into all of the pharmacies he got busted for. I was taken from my cell to a room where my new attorney was waiting to talk to me. Guess who was sitting there? None other than the same lawyer I had threatened to smack on the top of his head to make him shorter. Yeah, exactly, so I told him that he can't represent me for conflicts of interest because of our run-in with each other and me threatening him. But the court wouldn't hear it, because he was the only court-appointed *special* public defender in town. Well, I just gave up. But my cop buddy had made a deal with the courts and brought the chief state attorney to the court and got me out after a month. You know how that worked out—it was just after that when I got the 4 years sentence.

While I was in prison for 4 years, my girlfriend Kerry had gotten out. She got married and had 2 kids, all while I was in prison. But when I got out, we hooked up again. She told me that Bobby, the kid that told the court it was all my fault, kept asking her when I was getting out because he was worried about what was going to happen to him. Now, Kerry, Bobby, and I had all hung out with each other at my house. I knew Bobby before I knew Kerry, and we were all doing the scripts together.

Bobby died before I got out of prison. I heard he was a mess from Methadone and Heroin.

Kerry would repeatedly run away from her husband and run to me for a week, at the most, before I'd kick her out again, just like when we used to be together. Her multiple personalities were just too much for me to handle. Especially when I was trying to deal with my own mental distress from my marriage falling apart. A few years ago, Kerry came to live with me again. She asked me to bring her to Planned Parenthood for an abortion. She said she couldn't have another child by her husband, after three kids already and possession of none.

The very last time Kerry came over, she had had a tooth pulled. That was on a Wednesday. On the following Saturday, she was talking to her husband, and woke me up from a nap and asked me to take her home.

Her husband was seeing a girl, and she wanted to evaluate the situation. I said, fuck him and his new girl, but she persisted in having me bring her home. She went into the house, came back out a few minutes later, and said she thought she should stay because he was on the floor crying like a baby. I said, fuck him, but she said she would call me later for a ride back to my house. I knew better than that, but I got my piece of ass, so fuck her. I was used to her game. Now on that following Monday, I got up to go to work, driving a tractor-trailer delivering steel to NYC, but I saw I missed a call at 3 A.M. There was a message, and it was Kerry's husband, crying on the phone, saying that Kerry's heart wasn't strong enough and how she couldn't take it, and she was in the hospital, about 10 miles from my home town. While the guys were loading my truck, I told them I was going to the hospital to see what was going on. I got to the hospital and asked to see Kerry, and the nurses at the desk asked if I was family? I knew right then she wasn't doing well, or worse, so I told them that she lived with me. They asked me if I wanted to see her. Then I knew she was already dead. Eventually, I said, yeah, I want to see her, and I also wanted to talk to a detective. I walked into the room. She was lying on her back with a tube still in her mouth about 8 inches long. There was blood all around her mouth. She was bluish in color and seemed to be bloated. I had never seen a dead body before, so I didn't know what to expect. I could only say what the fuck to her and stroked her hair and walked out of the room.

Then I spoke to the detectives while they recorded me and I told them her husband killed her because of jealousy and what the situation had been over the previous week. Her husband asked me to be at the funeral. While I was there, her little sister told me that they'd keep me posted on the autopsy. Her husband said to me that she was throwing up a pinkish fluid all over the place before the ambulance came. A few months later, her sister called me and said that Kerry died from an infection from the tooth she had pulled the Wednesday before her death. The next week the dentist's office called me to see if she was going to be at her appointment the following day. All I said was no. The dentist should have never pulled an infected tooth to begin with. Supposed to wait until the infection was gone. That's why you wait.

—"getting my shit together"—

As I was approaching the end of my time forging prescriptions, I went through a big bin of garbage in the back of a pharmacy and found all kinds of patient records. Insurance info, what drugs they were taking, everything. I grabbed as much as I could carry. I kept seeing records with this drug I hadn't seen before. OxyContin. 10 mg, 20 mg, 40 mg. I started writing for Oxys. I would get 100 pills, 40 mg for $500 cash. I could turn that around for almost $2000 immediately without even opening the bottle. The 80 mg I would pay anywhere from $900 to $1,000 for 100 pills. I could turn that around for $3,500. Near the end of my forging "career," I made $36,000 in 6 weeks just from OxyContin.

By this time, I had gotten off the Methadone. I had a safe full of OxyContin, pints of Hycodan, pints of Tussionex—which is a more potent Hydrocodone syrup. We used to call it "Mother's Milk." It was very sweet. Then a buddy of mine turned me on to Duragesic patches. They were easily 100 times stronger than Morphine.

A year earlier, I had bought a Harley Davidson with the money I had made from OxyContin. I paid $15,000 in cash. A year and 1,000 miles later, I sold it for $10,000. All that money went to buying patches. $500 for 10 patches. I wasn't selling them, I used them. All of them. By this time, I was living at my mother's. Eventually, I violated my probation. They gave me a $10,000 bond. I had burned all my bridges; nobody would help. My friend at the state came to court, bringing some big shot from the chief state attorney's office. He said, Keith, you're gonna stay here for the month, and everything is going to be wiped clean when you get out. I said, Alright. I could hardly see, I was having seizures, hearing voices. Things were terrible at this point. It all came to a head. I stopped everything cold turkey. All the pills, the patches, even cigarettes.

I got out of jail and was getting my shit together. I knew a kid from the Methadone program that owed me money, and I went to collect. I still had some Xanax left in my glove compartment from before I went to jail. I saw a girl I knew, and she asked if I had any Xanax. I had no money, so I sold her 7 pills. Well, a police officer was stationed in the parking lot of the Methadone program and witnessed this transaction. She came over and pulled the girl out of the car. I could see them talking, and I saw her take a bottle of pills out of her purse and show it to the cop. The cop came over to my car, reached across me, and grabbed my bottle of Xanax. They said some things, but the only thing I heard was, You're under arrest. I went to court and appeared before the same judge I had seen before going away for a month. He's the one who set the conditions of my clean record. One of which was possessing no drugs for 2 months.

My dad was really sick at the time, and I saw my buddy from the state in court. I told him that my dad's going to die while I'm in prison, and he said, Oh, well. He had stuck his neck out for years, and it was time for me to pay the piper. I ended up getting 4 years, but in my state, non-violent criminals only serve half the time. They put me in a level 5 prison, the highest security. I remembered from years before, when I was 31 or 32, a drug control agent had told me, "There are only two outcomes for addiction. Death or jail." Well, here I was.

I look back and realize most of the people I did scripts with are dead. One kid I knew would rob pharmacies with a ski mask and pistol and demand what was in the safe. He ended up doing 20 years for armed bank robbery. I remember me and a couple of buddies decided we were going to rob a pharmacy. We drove around for a while until we found one. I went in to scope it out. There was a woman behind the counter, so I started to chit-chat with her. She told me about her son and other things. I went out and told my buddies it was cool. One buddy had a screwdriver, the other had a can of Mace and a big laundry bag. They ran in and yelled, "This is a robbery!" Someone yelled back, "No, it isn't!" to which they replied, "Yes, it is!"

They didn't even get a lot of drugs. The pharmacy wasn't stocked up. The girl behind the counter said, "Please don't kill me, I have a child." After we went home, I thought about the lady pleading for her life. That really ate at me. I ended up telling my friend at the state about what we did and asked where I should turn myself in. He kind of brushed it aside. But I insisted because it was eating at me. He told me the name of some state police officer for major crimes. I went there with my wife and figured it'd be routine. Give me a court date and send me on my way. Well, they slapped the cuffs on me and gave me a $75,000 bond.

—"how beautiful life is"—

I feel that this is the best part of my story. It's making me cry.

I've come to the conclusion that almost all of the people who are addicts are very intelligent, ultra-aware, and ultra-sensitive. They find temporary relief from all of life's stimuli through drugs. All addicts seem to suffer from some type of mental illness, whether depression, anxiety, multiple personalities, or manic depression. If you spend time with them, you see how one or two major crises in their lives shut them down and caused them to take refuge most quickly and efficiently to save what feels like their sanity. And doing it along with their friends. It's easier to take shelter with friends than with professionals. But it turns out to be the worst mistake, made while your brain is in a fight or flight mode for survival.

After my divorce, I found refuge in strip joints and became good friends with a lot of dancers. I was close to this one girl, Kris, who was very pretty but married to a hitman for the Angels. My buddy, who was with the statewide narcotics task force from in the '70s, infiltrated the Angels and was a prospect for them before he took them down. That's a whole other book. But he told me to be very careful, and if anyone came over to her house while I was there that had colors on (the Angels' vest), to leave. But I told him, fuck them. That's how much I was hurt by my wife cheating on me. But I went to prison, and when I got out, I ended up hanging out with hookers. Kind of like living my drug life through them, I'd drive them around while they got high. I had sympathy for them. I'd tell them that it only takes one bad stroke of luck and anyone could end up on the street.

I became a very trusted friend and confidant to some of them. I'd let them crash at my apartment if they had nowhere to go. I was fucking most of them, but after a while, I didn't get charged any money. I even brought a young Puerto Rican girl here to my mom's house for Xmas, 'cause otherwise, the girl was going to be alone in a hotel room. My son, my mother, the hooker, and I had Xmas dinner together. The girl brought Mom a gift, and Mom got her a gift. LOL. Yeah, I know, I'm fucking nuts, but I have a good heart, and so do most of the girls on the street.

I was with one girl who was 21 years old, I was 50, my son was older than she was. We got the apartment together that I lived in for seven years. She got a job, but later split. Then I hooked up with another gorgeous girl for two years. This girl was 20 years younger than me. (Oh, my poor mom and son.) She has a little girl that was a year old when we started dating. We broke up after three years. She was going to nursing school and straightened right out. One week after we split up, she was back out on the street. She got married but left the baby with her mother. I still see the baby, ten years old now and loves me. We go to the museum to see the dinosaurs. I buy her crafts to do and we come here to Mom's house. I don't want to disappear as her mother did—I feel a responsibility toward her.

This is how I have firsthand information about most drug addicts. Some crazy life, huh?

I would always stress to the girls how beautiful life is being clean. This one girl, Jess, who is the only one of the girls I still talk to, cried when I told her that they put me on narcotics when I had the surgery.

I would bring apples and fruit to the girls because they would spend every dime on Crack or Heroin. Just regular people who made terrible choices. I met a lot of their mothers and got to know them personally. I would urge the girls to get on the Methadone program so they wouldn't have to be out there doing what they were doing. Most of the time, Methadone wouldn't last long, and they would be back on the streets. It was as much of an addiction selling themselves as taking drugs. I figured it went hand in hand. Get picked up, that's the beginning of the high. Do their deed, second part of the high. Then cop the drugs, third part of the high. Then the high itself. Then the regret, and start all over again to squash the guilt of it all. Never ends.

—"happily married"—

As for girls buying pills from me, we would talk about the trade. I would sell pills to some girls that would sit down next to me at my and my wife's home and lean over and whisper that they'd suck my dick for 2 Percocet pills. Sad what drugs do to people. Other girls that I was sending into pharmacies would sit in the passenger seat with their legs open with no panties on.

But I never cheated on my wife with all the offers and deals from these girls. When you sell drugs, you're very popular with everyone, especially the girls who think you're an easy target. I would literally say to some of them that I was happily married. They'd look at me like I just fell out of the sky.

After my divorce, I was lost and didn't know what to do or where to go. I was alone after 20 years of marriage and very depressed and feeling lost. I had friends, but I had enjoyed being married and a homebody.

—"shadow on the wall"—

During the time I was living with my mother and father at their house, I was pretty much fucked up physically as well as mentally. I would stay up in my bedroom with my Fentanyl patches. I would eat tinned tuna fish from the can, drink creamed corn from the can, eat bags of Reese's peanut butter cups, and smoke cigarettes which Mom had forbidden me to do in the house.

This part of the story hurts for me to recall.

I would buy scented candles and burn them all day and night to mask the cigarette smoke. I would remake candles from the left-over candle wax and use the fringe from the blanket I had on my bed as wick. One night while letting the candle burn for heat and to disguise the cigarette smoke, I turned towards the wall with my back to the candle and TV. I opened my eyes and noticed a shadow flickering on the wall. I turned around and realized that my blankets were on fire, enough to cast a shadow on the wall.

After I had gotten out of prison, my mom and I were talking about when I was living there before I went to prison and she said that there were times when she didn't know if she and my dad would wake up the next morning because she feared I would light the house on fire. So sad the things that I put my family through.

I remember calling my mom from prison right after my father passed away and I told my mom that I might be able to TS (Transitional Service) out of prison to her house. She said that I wasn't welcome back to her home because of all the stress I had put her through before I went to prison. That hurt me because I had nobody to live with. To be able to get out, you need somebody to sign for your release, to be allowed to TS into someone's care and also to receive parole. I eventually did, after 30 months (out of a 4-year sentence). In my home state at the time, you were allowed to be paroled after ½ of the original sentence for a nonviolent crime, ¾ of your time if it was a violent crime. My sentence was a drug-related crime, so I was eligible for parole at 24 months. I was approved for release at 24 months, but I threatened a CO (corrections officer) so the parole board retracted my original parole. I had another hearing 5 months later and was eventually released after an extra 6 months in prison. And one other thing that the parole board stuck me with was an ankle bracelet or monitor with the condition that I was to be home from 6 P.M. to 6 A.M. which I was very fed up with because only violent criminals, rapists, gun crimes ... I never heard of an ankle bracelet for a drug conviction especially since I had to wear it for 3 months.

—"like a thief in the night"—

I hope people who read this book will take away a few vital lessons and suggestions, some of which may be life-altering; some for the better, perhaps some for the worse. I realize that any form of addiction is unhealthy—for everyone affected by the addict's life and choices.

One of the effects on the person addicted is the loss of the true feelings he is suppressing. Or that he can't find time to articulate to loved ones, friends, and people who he comes into contact with. Even if it's just a single contact. Addicts go through life fully engrossed in every second of their being. Worrying about the next fix, or being sick and wishing they had never got into the mess destroying their lives. To the unaware and nonaddicted public, the focus on getting high sounds selfish and self-centered. Maybe it is, but not to the addict who ended up in this terrible predicament.

Addiction comes up like a thief in the night. Without any warning. When it involves pharmaceutical opioids, it could happen to a person who never did any drugs their entire life. It can be the result of an automobile accident, long-term illness, back pain, migraine headaches. A person can become an addict without knowing that the drugs they are given are addictive or can easily be abused. And before they are aware of even a hint of the problem that might be festering within the brain ... boom! They've become addicted to a prescription drug. While some people can just go on with their lives, others want the doctor to prescribe more and more of the drug. If the doctor refuses, the patient feels wronged by the doctor. The doctor may think that the patient can't still be in pain and that the patient is just trying to scam him for more pills. The doctor is only human, and also has feelings, and may tell the patient to find another doctor. Often, the addict will do just that, find another doctor.

That patient may begin to "shop" for another doctor who will sympathize with the problems they might be suffering, whether real or psychosomatic. In all too many cases nowadays, the doctor just gives the patient the medication the patient desires, whether needed or not—for the money.

By 2017, the hammer had begun to come down on the doctors, to stop prescribing opioids in such large numbers, even in maintenance cases.

For example, I was recently at my pain specialist. I told her that I was not getting through the night without waking up in pain, and I asked the doctor to increase the dosage of my pain medication. She told me that she couldn't. That the state DCP was requiring doctors to bring patients down on dosage, and with some patients, bringing them off opioids entirely. That the DCP was coming up with different guidelines for prescribing opioids. They were frowning on prescribing opioids for bone pain unless you've had surgery. Also, she said there were quite a lot of other more effective medications. Why, I thought, didn't you go that route first and then prescribe opioids as a last resort? But I didn't say it out loud.

When I first started going to this pain clinic, you couldn't find room to stand up. Now there are only a couple of people in the waiting room. The state drug agency has put the word out that if you want to practice medicine in the state, cool it with over-prescribing opioids. Now that they have let the genie out of the bottle, people are being cut off cold-turkey without being taken down off the drugs slowly. I bet that 99% of doctors don't even think about patients becoming addicted. As long as they are no longer involved with the problem they started, and the state isn't on their backs, who cares? Then those same people, who might be your husband, wife, mother, father, sister, brother or child, who need to not feel like they are dying, start buying pills off of whoever has them for sale. If that can't be done, they are going to the people who have Heroin or anything else that will end the suffering. That is when you start seeing more and more overdoses and deaths. And it all may have started with one too many doctor visits. From a productive human being to another statistic. On the other side of the coin, most doctors don't know if their new patient is already a drug addict or prescription drug abuser. They only have the patient's word to go on.

As in my case. The clinic that I've been going to for a year now had me sign all kinds of paperwork, asking if I have or had ever been on pain medication and if I ever had a problem with abuse or addiction. My whole drug history. But I have a legitimate chronic pain condition. If I had been honest on the questionnaire, I would have been denied relief for the pain I experience. Now that is another problem for me and the surgeon, how to treat an addict with post-operative pain? And the surgeon is only responsible for 1 or 2 months of your pain following surgery, then you're told if you are still experiencing pain, you must go back to your regular practitioner for any more pain medication. Before recommending me to the surgeon, my doctor told me that he worried about the post-operative pain, and that he wasn't pleased with the way surgeons push the now opioid reliant patients back on to the primary physician. Which is what they did to my doctor, whom I deeply respect, and to me. Still, I do respect my surgeon.

For sure, I was negligent in not telling both of my doctors that I once had an addiction to opioids. I was afraid that they wouldn't prescribe them for the severe pain I was in before and after the surgery. I honestly believed that I would have power over the drugs this time because of all I had gone through before and in prison. I just didn't take it seriously enough. I thought I was wiser and had the mental ability to overcome any kind of addiction. At least this time. The pain was so intense before the surgery that I was taking up to 800 mg of Ibuprofen every 3 hours. This, while I was driving a tractor-trailer for 14 hours a day, and going straight to the chiropractor directly after work. Until I made my appointment for the surgery, I went without any opioids for the pain. But once I had the appointment, I asked my primary physician for something stronger to get me through until I had the surgery. After I had the surgery, I was prescribed 20 mg Oxycodone every 3 hours for the pain and 10 mg Valium 3 times a day. After 2 months, I was released by the surgeon to my primary physician to take me off the Oxycodone, or to continue using it. He wasn't comfortable with giving me any more Oxycodone. He said if I was still in pain that he could recommend a pain specialist, but he left the choice up to me. I chose the pain clinic.

—"Dexedrine"—

I remember when my young son was given a prescription for Dexedrine, 5 mg and 10 mg to treat ADHD. I had a problem with his pediatrician for prescribing this drug. So, I told the doctor about my own hassle with addiction. We discussed the prescription. He assured me that it had great potential to save my son from addiction because he wouldn't be looking for relief from the ADHD once he got older. Anything to help my child to not become an addict. This doctor had already prescribed Ritalin, but that didn't seem to work for my son. Therefore, it was Dexedrine.

Recently clean from Methadone, my wife was also taking Dexedrine. I only found that out because my son was missing pills from each prescription bottle. Of course, she denied stealing them. But they weren't just disappearing into thin air. And she had a bad track record from taking Percocet from me for many years. On top of that, she had also lost a treasonous amount of weight in a very brief time. She joined a gym, couldn't sit still, and wanted to go out every night, even during the workweek. I didn't know what was normal and what wasn't, because it had been a long time since I had gotten clean from drugs. I just thought it was a normal thing to have so much energy. Well, I was a fool for believing that she wasn't taking the pills from my son.

I had bought her a nice car so she wouldn't have to rush home after work every day, and I could go out to do the forged prescriptions every night. I preferred night time because I could hide my car more quickly if I needed to run from a pharmacy.

I was home one Saturday night—with depression and anxiety, as usual. My life was terrible. As far as socializing—I simply didn't. But my wife went out to a bar. Now the bars closed at 2 A.M. on the weekends, and I had gone to bed. Around 3 A.M., I started to get worried. There were no cell phones in the '90s, and I knew where she had gone to drink. She said she was going with her girlfriends from work. Anyway, she turned out not to be with the girls.

At that point, I went utterly downhill, mentally and physically. I was suffering from PTSD, according to my psychiatrist, who wanted to increase my Xanax dosage. I said no to that, I needed to deal with it.

About 8 months after this bar date, she sent me divorce papers. That's when I started going to strip joints almost every night. My son had stopped taking Dexedrine for his ADHD because it was making him feel weird. Instead of notifying his doctor, I would call in for refills without my son's knowledge, and I'd pick them up. Most of the strippers were using some sort of drugs, whether it was Cocaine or Speed, or Amphetamine (i.e., Dexedrine). I asked a couple of the girls if they wanted to buy some and, of course, they did. Every night I would be at the strip joint selling Dexedrine and Percocet.

I was The Man to the girls, and it helped me with my less than favorable self-image now that I was single. I became good friends with this really pretty blond-haired dancer. Besides being my client for the Dexedrine, she always wanted me to come over to her mom's house after work, as well as whenever she wasn't working. One night, one of the other girls asked me if I knew who she was and who she was married to. No, I didn't, and I didn't care. Well, they told me to read the name of the guy tattooed on her ass cheek. Yeah, so what? He was a very high-ranking biker in the Angels. I really didn't care and continued to go about my business with her. Another night I was on the phone with her, and her mother picked up the other phone in her house and said to me that I have to stop giving her daughter Dexedrine! I said that I didn't know what she was talking about, and the girl (the stripper) said, Yes, you do, Keith! Then the girl hung up, 'cause her mom told her to, and her mother proceeded to tell me that she (the stripper) was a very sick girl. I said, OK, and hung up the phone. About a year later, the girl called me and told me that she just had breast implants and wondered if I had any OxyContin for sale. We hooked up, and she said to me that she had broken up with the high-ranking biker, but had married the president of the NYC chapter of the same bike club! I never saw her again. She was a beautiful girl. I couldn't even take pictures of us together because she was the *property* of that particular club. Even she needed permission to use her own image for anything other than to promote her ass for money and stripper-related activities. All for money.

I couldn't use her name because of the people who she was affiliated with. Her tattoo read Danny.

I didn't want to get into the whole divorce thing. Still, I kept my wife from all of the bad things that I could, only our closest friends and some family ever knew that she got high, never mind being a drug addict. But as I write this, I still tend to protect her, mostly because of our son. I hope I haven't dragged her through the mud. I left out the part about how I caught her in the new car I had bought her… with a young man. I feel it explains the connection to the strippers in Florida and back home. I have to be honest about how and why I was acting as if I wasn't married.

—"the Narcan Challenge"—

My psychiatrist had a lot of pull. He was the head doctor for the Mental Health Center at the Ivy League college for 10 years, also the head man at a rehab facility for 10 years. Twenty years of mental health and drug addiction, he knew his way around. He was good friends with the guy who started the Methadone clinics in New York and my home state. He told me to get on Methadone. My wife and I were the first ones in the local clinic to get treated without being heroin addicts. People thought we were "lightweights" being addicted to pills, to painkillers.

Back then, they did what was called the Narcan Challenge. They would shoot you up with Narcan (Naloxone) to see if you got sick. Luckily, we didn't have to do that.

Coming soon:

Wanted: The #1 Opioid Prescription Forger & Doctor Shopper

True Stories of Surviving 20 Years of Opioid Addiction

☞ **PART II – The Dirt: Details & Documents** ☜

About the Author

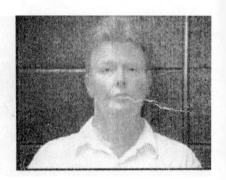

Inmate Number
0303566
Name(Last,First,Middle Init.)
LAPOINTE,KEITH
Date of Birth   Bond
12/29/1956   0010000
Height   Weight
5 ft **11** in   **250** lbs

These are true stories—adventures and misadventures—of an opioid drugs addict. Keith "Woody" LaPointe survived 20 years of drug use, incarceration (with a *cold-turkey withdrawal*), and return to the outside world of meaningful family living and gainful employment. Twenty years of being the **#1 doctor-shopper and prescription forger***. And then, following an accident, a life-threatening relapse. Once again, back to the incredibly difficult work of rehabilitation.

*As documented in a local ABC-affiliate TV news special and as known to the state Department of Consumer Protection, Drug Control Division [DCP].

R <u>PART II – The Dirt: Details & Documents</u>

Made in United States
North Haven, CT
05 September 2023